Student Study Guide

to accompany

DISCOVERING NUTRITION

Second Edition

Paul Insel
Stanford University

R. Elaine Turner, RD
University of Florida

Don Ross
California Institute of Human Nutrition

JONES AND BARTLETT PUBLISHERS
Sudbury, Massachusetts
BOSTON TORONTO LONDON SINGAPORE

World Headquarters
Jones and Bartlett Publishers
40 Tall Pine Drive
Sudbury, MA 01776
978-443-5000
info@jbpub.com

Jones and Bartlett Publishers Canada
6339 Ormindale Way
Mississauga, Ontario L5V 1J2
CANADA

Jones and Bartlett Publishers International
Barb House, Barb Mews
London W6 7PA
UK

Jones and Bartlett's books and products are available through most bookstores and online booksellers. To contact Jones and Bartlett Publishers directly, call 800-832-0034, fax 978-443-8000, or visit our website, www.jbpub.com.

Substantial discounts on bulk quantities of Jones and Bartlett's publications are available to corporations, professional associations, and other qualified organizations. For details and specific discount information, contact the special sales department at Jones and Bartlett via the above contact information or send an email to specialsales@jbpub.com.

ISBN-13: 978-0-7637-3899-0
ISBN-10: 0-7637-3899-9

Production Credits
Acquisitions Editor: Jacqueline Mark-Geraci
Senior Production Editor: Julie C. Bolduc
Associate Editor: Nicole L. Quinn
Editorial Assistant: Amy L. Flagg
Associate Marketing Manager: Wendy Thayer
Manufacturing Buyer: Therese Connell
Composition: Shawn Girsberger
Cover Design: Anne Spencer
Cover Image: Stephen Ausmus/Agricultural Research Service/USDA
Printing and Binding: Courier Stoughton
Cover Printing: Courier Stoughton

6048

Printed in the United States of America
10 09 08 07 06 10 9 8 7 6 5 4 3 2

Contents

Introduction

The topic of nutrition is both important and complex. For some students, this course is required to fulfill degree requirements for graduation; others choose this as an elective. All students can benefit from the volume of information covered in a course in nutrition.

In this course and text, you will discover valuable information about nutrition that may affect diet decisions in your own life. You will learn about vitamins, minerals, fats, and proteins and the benefits of a healthful diet. You will also learn about government policies to thwart hunger and the effects of the environment on what you eat. This course and text will provide you with the knowledge needed to choose a nutritiously rewarding diet and to lead a healthier life. This may well be the most personally useful course you take in your academic career. The knowledge gained in this course can both protect and enhance your life.

This study guide is designed to help you organize and reinforce your learning about the nutrition topics covered in the *Discovering Nutrition*, Second Edition text. The following features can be found in each chapter:

- **Key Terms** Provide definitions for the chapter's glossary terms.
- **Fill-in-the-Blanks** Using glossary terms from the chapter, complete each sentence to test your knowledge of some of the chapter's key ideas.
- **Fill-in-the-Blank Summaries** After you read the chapter, use this feature to test and refresh your memory of the topics covered.
- **Student Note-Taking Guide** This feature covers the key points in your book. It helps you to have organized notes, which is essential at exam time and when doing assignments.
- **Answers to Study Guide questions** can be found on the *Discovering Nutrition*, Second Edition website: http://nutrition.jbpub.com/discovering.

Student Note-Taking Guide

In addition to many of the above components, which will help you understand chapter content by testing and reviewing key concepts and terms, this study guide also serves as a Student Note-Taking Guide, which will help you learn by providing a structure to your notes. The Student Note-Taking Guide component is located directly after the Fill-in-the-Blank Summaries in each chapter and contains the full set of PowerPoint slides that accompany your textbook as well as space next to each slide for you to jot down the terms and concepts that you feel are most important to each lecture.

The Student Note-Taking Guide is your partner and guide in note-taking. If your instructor is using the PowerPoint slides that accompany the text, this guide will save you from having to write down everything that is on the slides. Do the assigned reading, listen in lecture, follow the key points your instructor makes, and write down meaningful notes. Your note-taking guide is the perfect place to write down questions that you want to ask your professor later or reminders to yourself to go back and study a certain concept again to make sure you really got it.

For more information on the most effective note-taking methods that will save you both time and effort when reviewing for exams, see the section on Note-Taking Tips directly following this Introduction.

Once the Student Note-Taking Guide component of this Study Guide has helped to organize and simplify your notes on each chapter, the exercises in the remaining sections of the Study Guide will test how well you have mastered the material. Your ability to easily locate the important concepts of a recent lecture and test yourself on the most important points and terminology will prove to be essential at exam time.

This Study Guide is a valuable resource. You've found a wonderful study partner!

Note-Taking Tips

1. It is easier to take notes if you are not hearing the information for the first time. Read the chapter or the material that is about to be discussed before class. This will help you to anticipate what will be said in class, and have an idea of what to write down. It will also help to read over your notes from the last class. This way you can avoid having to spend the first few minutes of class trying to remember where you left off last time.

2. Don't waste your time trying to write down everything that your professor says. Instead, listen closely and only write down the important points. Review these important points after class to help remind you of related points that were made during the lecture.

3. If the class discussion takes a spontaneous turn, pay attention and participate in the discussion. Only take notes on the conclusions that are relevant to the lecture.

4. Emphasize main points in your notes. You may want to use a highlighter, special notation (asterisks, exclamation points), format (circle, underline), or placement on the page (indented, bulleted). You will find that when you try to recall these points, you will be able to actually picture them on the page.

5. Be sure to copy down word-for-word specific formulas, laws, and theories.

6. Hearing something repeated, stressed, or summed up can be a signal that it is an important concept to understand.

7. Organize handouts, study guides, and exams in your notebook along with your lecture notes. It may be helpful to use a three-ring binder, so that you can insert pages wherever you need to.

8. When taking notes, you might find it helpful to leave a wide margin on all four sides of the page. Doing this allows you to note names, dates, definitions, etc. for easy access and studying later. It may also be helpful to make notes of questions you want to ask your professor about or research later, ideas or relationships that you want to explore more on your own, or concepts that you don't fully understand.

9. It is best to maintain a separate notebook for each class. Labeling and dating your notes can be helpful when you need to look up information from previous lectures.

10. Make your notes legible, and take notes directly in your notebook. Chances are you won't recopy them no matter how noble your intentions. Spend the time you would have spent recopying the notes studying them instead, drawing conclusions and making connections that you didn't have time for in class.

11. Look over your notes after class while the lecture is still fresh in your mind. Fix illegible items and clarify anything you don't understand. Do this again right before the next class.

CHAPTER 1

Food Choices: Nutrients and Nourishment

◎ Chapter Outline

The chapter outline provides you with an organizational guide to the topics and ideas presented in this chapter of the text.

Why Do We Eat the Way We Do?
- Sensory Influences: Taste, Texture, and Smell
- Cognitive Influences
- Environmental Influences
- The American Diet

Introducing the Nutrients
- Definition of Nutrients
- Carbohydrates
- Lipids
- Proteins
- Vitamins
- Minerals
- Water
- Nutrients and Energy
- Energy in Foods
- Obesity: A Public Health Crisis

Applying the Scientific Process to Nutrition
- Epidemiological Studies
- Animal Studies
- Cell Culture Studies
- Human Studies
- More on the Placebo Effect

From Research Study to Headline
- Peer Review of Experimental Results
- Sorting Facts and Fallacies in the Media

◎ Key Terms

Define the following terms.

1. **antioxidant** ______________________________
2. **case control study** ______________________________
3. **double-blind study** ______________________________
4. **flavor** ______________________________
5. **inorganic** ______________________________

6. **neophobia** ______________________________

7. **pica** ______________________________

8. **umami** ______________________________

9. **social facilitation** ______________________________

10. **placebo** ______________________________

11. **circulation** ______________________________

12. **experimental group** ______________________________

13. **triglycerides** ______________________________

14. **minerals** ______________________________

15. **peer review** ______________________________

16. **micronutrients** ______________________________

17. **phytochemicals** ______________________________

18. **organic** ______________________________

19. **nutrients** ______________________________

20. **legumes** ______________________________

Fill-in-the-Blank

1. Organic compounds that function as the building blocks of protein are ____________________.
2. Connections, co-occurring more frequently than can be explained by chance or coincidence, but without a proven cause are called ____________________.
3. A ____________________ is a scientist's "educated guess" to explain phenomenon.
4. ____________________ is the science of foods and their components (nutrients and other substances) including the relationships to health and disease (actions, interactions, and balances); processes within the body (ingestion, digestion, absorption, transport, functions, and disposal of end products); and the social, economic, cultural, and psychological implications of eating.
5. The capacity to do work is ____________________.
6. ____________________ are organic compounds necessary for reproduction, growth, and maintenance of the body. They are required in minuscule amounts.
7. Substances that must be obtained in the diet because the body either cannot make them or cannot make adequate amounts of them are ____________________.
8. Nutrients, such as carbohydrate, fat, or protein, that are needed in relatively large amounts in the diet are ____________________.

9. A ______________________ is a set of people used as a standard of comparison to the experimental group. The people in this group have characteristics similar to those in the experimental group and are selected at random.

10. ______________________ is the science of determining the incidence and distribution of diseases in different populations.

11. The general term for energy in food, used synonymously with the term energy, is ______________________ ______________________.

12. ______________________ are compounds, including sugars, starches, and dietary fibers, that usually have the general chemical formula $(CH_2O)_n$, where n represents the number of CH_2O units in the molecule.

13. ______________________ are tests to examine the validity of a hypothesis.

14. Food energy is measured in ______________________.

15. ______________________ are present in the body and required in the diet in relatively small amounts compared with major minerals. Also known as microminerals.

16. ______________________ are large, complex compounds consisting of many amino acids connected in varying sequences and forming unique shapes.

17. ______________________ are chemical messengers that are secreted into the blood by one tissue and act on cells in another part of the body.

18. A physical or emotional change that is not due to properties of an administered substance and that reflects participants' expectations is called ______________________.

19. Major minerals required in the diet and present in the body in large amounts are ______________________ ______________________.

20. ______________________ is the name for a group of fat-soluble compounds that includes triglycerides, sterols, and phospholipids.

◎ Fill-in-the-Blank Summaries

Why Do We Eat the Way We Do?

Pauline is a three-year-old child who will only eat bananas and PBJ. Her mother, Meg, is frustrated because she will not try anything new. Pauline is exhibiting characteristics of ______________________ ______________.

Because Meg is an adult and her tastes have matured, she has a greater appreciation for the ____________ ________________________ and texture of different foods. She loves the sensation of ____________ ________________________, the Japanese term that describes the taste produced by the amino acid ____. Meg tries hard to control her weight throughout the year, but like most Americans, she tends to gain weight around the holidays when she attends many family parties. The phenomenon that describes why Meg eats more at these functions is called ________ ________________.

Introducing the Nutrients

Food is a mixture of chemicals of which some are essential for normal body function. These essential chemicals are called ____. Carbohydrate, fat, and protein are all needed in relatively large amounts in the diet and are therefore classified as ______________ ________________________. Vitamins and minerals are classified as ________________________, as they are needed in relatively small amounts in the diet. Nutrients are composed of organic compounds that contain ________________________ and inorganic compounds that do not contain this element. Nonessential substances in plants that may possess health-protective effects are referred to as ________ ____________________________. These "plant chemicals" have important health functions which may reduce risk for heart disease and cancer.

A ______________________________ is a nutrient made of carbon, hydrogen and oxygen and is a major fuel source for the body. The term lipids refers to substances such as fats and oils, but also to fat-like substances in foods such as ________________________________ and phospholipids. Proteins are organic compounds made of smaller building blocks called ____________________________________. ______________________________ are organic compounds that contain carbon, hydrogen, and possibly nitrogen, oxygen, phosphorus, sulfur, and other elements. ____________________________ are simple inorganic substances that have structural and regulatory roles. Macrominerals are major minerals required by the body in relatively large quantities. Microminerals (or trace minerals) are required in the diet in relatively small amounts.

Notes

Discovering
Nutrition
Second Edition Paul Insel R. Elaine Turner Don Ross

Food Choices:
Nutrients and Nourishment

Chapter 1

Influences on Food Choices

- Sensory
  - Taste
    - Sweet, sour, bitter, salty
    - Umami
  - Smell
  - Texture

Influences on Food Choices

- Cognitive
  - Habits
  - Comfort/discomfort foods
  - Cravings
  - Advertising
  - Social factors
  - Nutritional value
  - Health beliefs

Notes

Influences on Food Choices

- Environment
  - Economic factors
  - Lifestyle
  - Culture
    - Religion
  - "American diet"

Photo © PhotoDisc

Introducing the Nutrients

- Definition of nutrients
  - Food = mixture of chemicals
  - Essential chemicals = nutrients

Introducing the Nutrients

Lipids
Vitamins
Water
Carbohydrates
Minerals
Proteins

- Six classes of nutrients
  - Carbohydrates
  - Lipids (fats and oils)
  - Proteins
  - Vitamins
  - Minerals
  - Water

Introducing the Nutrients

- Other chemicals in food
  - Flavors and colors
  - Caffeine
  - Phytochemicals

Introducing the Nutrients

- General functions of nutrients
  - Supply energy
    - Carbohydrates, lipids, proteins
  - Contribute to cell and body structure
  - Regulate body processes

Introducing the Nutrients

- Classifications of nutrients
  - Macronutrients
    - Carbohydrates, lipids, proteins
  - Micronutrients
    - Vitamins, minerals
  - Organic (contain carbon)
    - Carbohydrates, lipids, proteins, vitamins
  - Inorganic
    - Minerals, water

Notes

Notes

Introducing the Nutrients

- Carbohydrates
  - Sugars and starches
  - Functions
    - Energy source
  - Food sources
    - Grains
    - Vegetables
    - Fruits
    - Dairy products

Photo © PhotoDisc

Introducing the Nutrients

- Lipids
  - Triglycerides (fats and oils), cholesterol and phospholipids
  - Functions
    - Energy source, structure, regulation
  - Food sources
    - Fats and oils
    - Meats
    - Dairy products

Photo © PhotoDisc

Introducing the Nutrients

- Proteins
  - Made of amino acids
  - Functions
    - Energy source, structure, regulation
  - Food sources
    - Meats
    - Dairy products
    - Legumes, vegetables, grains

Photo © PhotoDisc

Introducing the Nutrients

- Vitamins
  - Fat-soluble
    - A, D, E, K
  - Water-soluble
    - B vitamins, vitamin C
  - Functions
    - Regulation
  - Food sources
    - All food groups

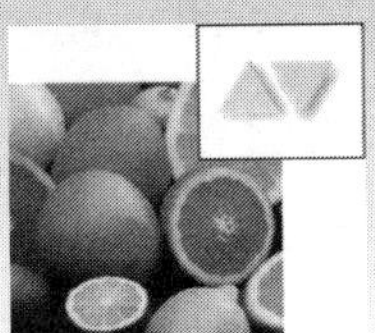

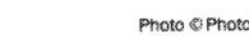

Photo © PhotoDisc

Introducing the Nutrients

- Minerals
  - Macrominerals and trace minerals
  - Functions
    - Structure, regulation
  - Food sources
    - All food groups

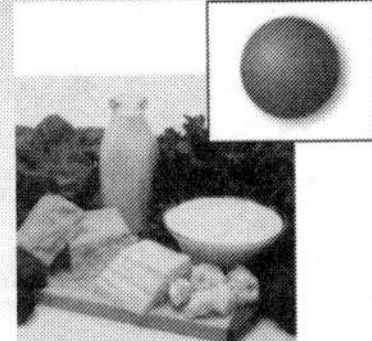

Photo © PhotoDisc

Introducing the Nutrients

- Water
  - Most important nutrient
  - Functions
    - Structure, regulation
  - Food sources
    - Beverages
    - Foods

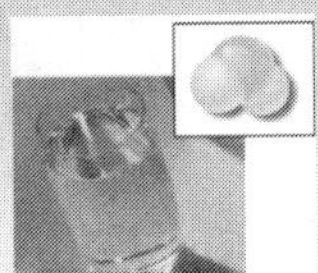

Photo © PhotoDisc

Notes

Notes

Introducing the Nutrients

- Energy in foods
  - Measured in kilocalories (kcal)

Introducing the Nutrients

- Obesity: public health crisis
  - 65% of U.S. adults are overweight or obese
  - Increases health risks
    - Type 2 diabetes
    - Cardiovascular diseases
    - Cancer
    - Gallbladder disease

Introducing the Nutrients

- Obesity: public health objectives
  - Reduce prevalence of obesity to 15%
  - Factors that influence obesity
    - Behavior
    - Environment
    - Genetics

Notes

Applying the Scientific Process to Nutrition

- Scientific method (see Figure 1.11, p. 20)
  - Observation
  - Hypothesis
  - Experimentation
  - Publication
  - Further experimentation
  - Theory

Applying the Scientific Process to Nutrition

- Types of studies
  - Epidemiological
  - Animal
  - Cell culture
  - Human
    - Case control
    - Clinical trial

From Research Study to Headline

- Peer review of experimental results
  - Scientific publication
- Media publication
  - Sorting facts and fallacies
  - Finding reliable sources

CHAPTER 2

Nutrition Guidelines: Tools for a Healthful Diet

Chapter Outline

The chapter outline provides you with an organizational guide to the topics and ideas presented in this chapter of the text.

Linking Nutrients, Foods, and Health
- The Continuum of Nutritional Status
- Moderation, Variety, and Balance: Words to the Wise

Dietary Guidelines
- *Dietary Guidelines for Americans*
- Using the Guidelines
- *Canada's Guidelines for Healthy Eating*

Food Groups and Food Guides
- A Brief History of Food Group Plans
- The USDA Food Guide Pyramid
- *Canada's Food Guide to Healthy Living*
- Using MyPyramid or *Canada's Food Guide* in Diet Planning

Exchange Lists

Recommendations for Nutrient Intake: The DRIs
- Understanding Dietary Standards
- A Brief History of Dietary Standards
- Dietary Reference Intakes

Food Labels
- Ingredients and Other Basic Information
- Nutrition Facts Panel
- Daily Values
- Nutrient Content Claims
- Health Claims
- Qualified Health Claims
- Structure/Function Claims
- Using Labels to Make Healthful Food Choices

Key Terms

Define the following terms.

1. **food groups** ______________________________
2. **enrich** ______________________________
3. **overnutrition** ______________________________
4. **Tolerable Upper Intake Levels (ULs)** ______________________________
5. **requirement** ______________________________

6. **U.S. Department of Health and Human Services (DHHS)** ______________________________

____

7. **Exchange Lists for Meal Planning** ______________________________

8. **Recommended Dietary Allowances (RDAs)** ______________________________

9. **Recommended Nutrient Intakes (RNIs)** ______________________________

10. **Estimated Energy Requirement (EER)** ______________________________

11. **dietary standards** ______________________________

12. **fortify** ______________________________

13. **Acceptable Macronutrient Distribution Ranges (AMDRs)** ______________________________

____

14. **Statement of Identity** ______________________________

15. **undernutrition** ______________________________

16. **Dietary Reference Intakes (DRIs)** ______________________________

◎ Fill-in-the-Blank

1. The intake value that meets the estimated nutrient needs of 50 percent of individuals in a specific life-stage and gender group is the ______________________________.

2. Recommendations to help Canadians select foods to meet energy and nutrient needs while reducing risk of chronic disease can be found in ______________________________.

3. The ______________________________ is an amendment to the Food, Drug, and Cosmetic Act of 1938. It made major changes to the content and scope of the nutrition label and to other elements of food labels. Final regulations were published in 1993 and went into effect in 1994.

4. The foundation of federal nutrition policy, the ______________________________ ______________________________, are jointly developed by the U.S. Department of Agriculture (USDA) and the Department of Health and Human Services (DHHS). These science-based guidelines are intended to reduce the number of Americans who develop chronic diseases such as hypertension, diabetes, cardiovascular disease, obesity, and alcoholism.

5. ______________________________ describe the level of a nutrient or dietary substance in a product, using terms such as good source, high, or free.

6. The federal agency responsible for assuring that foods sold in the United States (except for eggs, poultry, and meat) are safe, wholesome, and labeled properly is the ______________________________

________________________. This agency sets standards for the composition of some foods, inspects food plants, and monitors imported foods. It is part of the Public Health Services, a component of the U.S. Department of Health and Human Services (DHHS).

7. Food Labels are required by law on virtually all packaged foods and must include the following five requirements:

(1) ____

(2) ____

(3) ____

(4) ____

(5) ____

8. Any statement that associates a food or a substance in a food with a disease or health-related condition is a ________________________. The ________________________ ________________________ authorizes these.

9. ________________________ is an educational tool that translates the principles of the *2005 Dietary Guidelines for Americans* and other nutritional standards to help consumers in making healthier food and physical activity choices.

10. ________________________ include key messages that are based on the 1990 Nutrition Recommendations for Canadians and provide positive, action-oriented, scientifically accurate eating advice to Canadians.

11. ________________________ are a portion of the food label that states the content of selected nutrients in a food in a standard way prescribed by the Food and Drug Administration. By law, these must appear on nearly all processed food products in the United States.

12. The ________________________ is a graphic representation of USDA dietary guidelines; it has now been replaced by ________________________.

13. ________________________ are a single set of nutrient intake standards developed by the Food and Drug Administration to represent the needs of the "typical" consumer and are used as standards for expressing nutrient content on food labels.

14. The ________________________ monitors the production of eggs, poultry, and meat for adherence to standards of quality and wholesomeness. The agency also provides public nutrition education, performs nutrition research, and administers the WIC program.

15. The ________________________________ is responsible for assembling the group of nutrition scientists who review available scientific data to determine appropriate intake levels of the known essential nutrients.

16. ________________________________ are statements that may claim a benefit related to a nutrient-deficiency disease or describe the role of a nutrient or dietary ingredient intended to affect a structure or function in humans.

17. A set of scientific statements that provide guidance to Canadians for a dietary pattern that will supply recommended amounts of all essential nutrients while reducing the risk of chronic disease is the ________________________________.

18. ________________________________ is the nutrient intake that appears to sustain a defined nutritional state or some other indicator of health (e.g., growth rate or normal circulating nutrient values) in a specific population or subgroup. This is used when there is insufficient scientific evidence to establish an ________________________________.

◎ Fill-in-the-Blank Summaries

Dietary Guidelines

The USDA and ________________________ released some of the first general goals relating to nutrient intake and diet composition. The ____________________ promote food and lifestyle choices that reduce the risk for chronic disease and promote the basic principles of balance, variety, and moderation. Dietary standards are recommendations that tell us how much of each nutrient we need in our diets. The ___________________________ were originally developed for military purposes and are set at a level which generally meets the needs of almost all individuals. New dietary standards, the ___________________________, focus on optimal rather than adequate nutrition. Well before World War II, ________________________ were used in nutrition education to illustrate the proper combination of foods in a healthful diet. The USDA has now in 2005 introduced ________________ to provide a visual representation of the *Dietary Guidelines for Americans*. Another diet planning tool, the ________________________________, provides a guide for foods based on consistent levels of energy and carbohydrates. A third diet planning tool, the Food Label, provides a statement of identity, net contents, manufacturer information, a list of ingredients and nutrition information which assists consumers when making decisions at the grocery store. Information pertaining to ______________

__________ is located at the top of the Nutrition Facts label. For a label to read "calorie free" it must contain less than ______________ calories.

Linking Nutrients, Foods, and Health

Nutritional health involves obtaining all of the nutrients in amounts needed to support body processes. If someone has poor health due to inadequate intake of nutrients over time, this is referred to as ________________________________. Consuming too much food can be detrimental as well. ___________________________________ is the chronic consumption of more than is necessary for good health and can lead to chronic diseases. The USDA __________________________________ ____ illustrates the basic concepts of variety moderation, proportionality, physical activity, gradual improvement, and ____ to help Americans make healthy food choices and be active each day. Your diet is balanced if the amount of _______________ ________________________________ you take in is equal to the amount of energy you spend in daily activities and exercise.

Notes

Discovering
Nutrition
Second Edition Paul Insel R. Elaine Turner Don Ross

Nutrition Guidelines:
Tools for a Healthful Diet

Chapter 2

Linking Nutrients, Foods, and Health

- Continuum of nutritional status
  - Undernutrition
  - Good health
  - Overnutrition

Linking Nutrients, Foods, and Health

- Choosing a healthful diet
  - Moderation
  - Variety
  - Balance

Dietary Guidelines

- *Dietary Guidelines for Americans* (2005)
  - Science-based advice
  - Promote health, reduce chronic disease risk

Dietary Guidelines

- *Dietary Guidelines for Americans*
  - Adequate nutrients within calorie needs
  - Weight management
  - Physical activity
  - Food groups to encourage
    - Fruits, vegetables, whole grains, low-fat milk

Dietary Guidelines

- *Dietary Guidelines for Americans*
  - Fats
    - Limit total fat, saturated fat, *trans* fat, cholesterol
  - Carbohydrates
    - Limit added sugar; eat more whole grains
  - Sodium and potassium
  - Alcoholic beverages
  - Food safety

Notes

Notes

Dietary Guidelines

- *Canada's Guidelines for Healthy Eating*
  - Eat a variety of foods
  - Emphasize grains, vegetables, fruits
  - Choose lower-fat dairy, leaner meats
  - Achieve and maintain healthy weight through exercise and healthy eating
  - Limit salt, alcohol, caffeine

Food Groups and Food Guides

- History of Food Guides
  - Basic Four
  - USDA Food Guide Pyramid

MyPyramid

GRAINS | VEGETABLES | FRUITS | MILK | MEAT & BEANS

Source: USDA

MyPyramid

- Basic concepts
  - Variety
  - Moderation
  - Proportionality
  - Physical activity
  - Gradual improvement
  - Personalization

Exchange Lists

- Meal planning for people with diabetes
- Foods grouped by macronutrient content
  - Starches
  - Fruits
  - Milks
  - Other carbohydrates
  - Vegetables
  - Meats and meat substitutes
  - Fats
  - See Appendix B

Recommendations for Nutrient Intake

- Dietary Reference Intakes (DRIs)
  - Recommendations for nutrient intake
  - Developed by the Food and Nutrition Board
  - Apply to healthy people in the United States and Canada
  - Four basic elements

Notes

Notes

Dietary Reference Intakes (DRIs)

- Estimated Average Requirement (EAR)
  - Amount that meets the nutrient requirements of 50% of people in a life-stage and gender group
  - Based on functional indicator of optimal health

Meets the nutrient needs of 50% of a particular population
EAR
Number of people
Nutrient intake
ESTIMATED AVERAGE REQUIREMENT

Dietary Reference Intakes (DRIs)

- Recommended Dietary Allowance (RDA)
- Amount that meets the needs of most people in a life-state and gender group

Meets the nutrient needs of 97-98% of a particular population
RDA
Number of people
Nutrient intake
RECOMMENDED DIETARY ALLOWANCE

Dietary Reference Intakes (DRIs)

- Adequate Intake (AI)
  - Amount thought to be adequate for most people
  - AI is used when EAR and RDA can't be determined
- Tolerable Upper Intake Level (UL)
  - Intake above the UL can be harmful

ADEQUATE INTAKE
TOLERABLE UPPER INTAKE LEVEL

Dietary Reference Intakes (DRIs)

- Estimated Energy Requirement (EER)
  - Energy intake needed for energy balance
- Acceptable Macronutrient Distribution Range (AMDR)
  - Recommended balance of energy sources

Dietary Reference Intakes (DRIs)

- Using the DRIs
  - Population groups
    - Assess adequacy of intake
    - Plan diets
    - Set policy and guidelines
  - Individuals
    - Use RDA and AI as target levels for intake
    - Avoid intake greater than the UL

Food Labels

- Mandatory information on food labels
  - Statement of identity
  - Net contents of the package
  - Name and address of manufacturer, packer, and distributor
  - List of ingredients
    - Listed in descending order by weight
  - Nutrition information

Notes

Notes

Food Labels

- Nutrition Facts panel
  - Standard format

Nutrition Facts
Serving Size: 1 slice (34g/1.2 oz)
Servings Per Container: 20

Amount Per Serving	
Calories 90 Calories from fat 10	
	% Daily Value*
Total Fat 1g	2%
Saturated Fat 0g	1%
Trans Fat 0g	
Cholesterol 0mg	0%
Sodium 160mg	7%
Total Carbohydrate 15g	5%
Dietary Fiber 2g	8%
Sugars 2g	
Protein 4g	
Vitamin A 0% • Vitamin C 0%	
Calcium 0% • Iron 4%	

* Percent Daily Values are based on a 2,000 calorie diet. Your daily values may be higher or lower depending on your calorie needs:

	Calories:	2,000	2,500
Total Fat	Less Than	65g	80g
Sat Fat	Less Than	20g	25g
Cholesterol	Less Than	300mg	300mg
Sodium	Less Than	2,400mg	2,400mg
Total Carbohydrate		300g	375g
Dietary Fiber		25g	30g

Calories per gram:
Fat 9 • Carbohydrate 4 • Protein 4

Food Labels

- Daily Values
  - Compare amount in one serving to amount recommended for daily consumption
- Nutrient content claims
  - Descriptive terms (e.g., low fat, high fiber)
  - Defined by FDA (see pages 56–57)

Food Labels

- Health claims
  - Link one or more dietary components to reduced risk of disease
  - Must be supported by scientific evidence
  - Approved by FDA (see pages 57–58)
- Structure/function claims
  - Describe potential effects on body structure or function

CHAPTER 3

Complementary Nutrition: Functional Foods and Dietary Supplements

The chapter outline provides you with an organizational guide to the topics and ideas presented in this chapter of the text.

Functional Foods
- Phytochemicals Make Foods Functional
- Foods Enhanced with Functional Ingredients
- Regulatory Issues for Functional Foods

Food Additives
- Regulation by the FDA
- Delaney Clause
- Additives in Functional Foods

Claims for Functional Foods
- Structure/Function Claims for Functional Foods

Strategies for Functional Food Use

Dietary Supplements: Vitamins and Minerals
- Moderate Supplementation
- Megadoses in Conventional Medical Management
- Megadosing Beyond Conventional Medicine: Orthomolecular Nutrition
- Drawbacks of Megadoses

Dietary Supplements: Natural Health Products
- Helpful Herbs, Harmful Herbs
- Other Dietary Supplements

Dietary Supplements in the Marketplace
- The FTC and Supplement Advertising
- The FDA and Supplement Regulation
- Supplement Labels
- Canadian Regulations
- Choosing Dietary Supplements
- Fraudulent Products

Complementary and Alternative Medicine
- Where Does Nutrition Fit In?
- Special Diets, Food Restrictions, and Food Prescriptions

Key Terms

Define the following terms.

1. **bioavailability** ______________________________

2. **functional food** ______________________________

3. **dietary supplements** ______________________________

4. **color additive** ______________________________

5. **lycopene** ______________________________

6. **isoflavones** ______________________________

7. **Generally Recognized as Safe (GRAS)** ______________________________

8. **complementary and alternative medicine (CAM)** ______________________________

9. **macrobiotic diet** ______________________________

10. **prior-sanctioned substance** ______________________________

11. **multilevel marketing** ______________________________

12. **bioflavonoids** ______________________________

13. **direct additives** ______________________________

◎ Fill-in-the-Blank

1. The part of the 1960 Color Additives amendment to the Federal Food, Drug, and Cosmetic Act that bars the FDA from approving any products shown in laboratory tests to cause cancer is the ______________________________.

2. Established in 1820, ______________________________ is a voluntary, not-for-profit health care organization that sets quality standards for a range of health care products.

3. The ______________________________ is an NIH organization established to stimulate, develop, and support objective scientific research on complementary and alternative medicine for the benefit of the public.

4. ______________________________ are short-lived, highly reactive chemicals often derived from oxygen-containing compounds, which can have detrimental effects on cells, especially DNA and cell membranes.

5. Substances that become part of the food in trace amounts due to its packaging, storage, or other handling are ______________________________.

6. Conditions that result in imperfect, inadequate, or otherwise disordered gastrointestinal absorption are ______________________________.

7. Doses of a nutrient that are 10 or more times the recommended amount are called ______________________________.

8. The content label that must appear on all dietary supplements is called the ______________________________.

9. The ______________________________ regulates dietary supplements.

10. ________________________ is the therapeutic use of herbs and other plants to promote health and treat disease. It is also called ____________.

11. ________________________ involves the preventive or therapeutic use of high-dose vitamins to treat disease.

12. ________________________ are a family of more than 25,000 molecules found in chromosomes, nucleoli, mitochondria, and the cytoplasm of cells.

13. Substances added to food to perform various functions, such as adding color or flavor, replacing sugar or fat, improving nutritional content, or improving texture or shelf life are ________________ ________________.

◎ Fill-in-the-Blank Summaries

Functional Foods

A ________________________ is widely considered a food that may provide health beyond basic nutrition. Functional foods get their health-promoting properties from naturally occurring compounds that are not considered nutrients but are called ________________ ______. A vitamin is a food substance essential for health. Phytochemicals, in contrast, are substances in plants that may protect our good health, even though they ________________. Phytochemicals include thousands of compounds, pigments, and natural antioxidants, many of which are associated with protection from heart disease, hypertension, cancer, and ____________ ________________. Phytochemicals work to prevent cancer by neutralizing ________ ________________ and by modifying the way hormones affect the body. Free radicals are continually produced in our cells and over time can result in damage to ________________ ______ and other important cell structures.

Food Additives

Food additives work in many ways to give us safe, plentiful, varied, and relatively inexpensive food. Food additives are use for many reasons; these include improving product quality, maintaining freshness, and ________________. Food additives can either be direct or indirect. ____________ ____________ are added to food for a specific reason. ________________ are substances that unintentionally become part of the food in trace amounts. The ____________ ________ decides whether to approve the additive and determines that types of foods that may contain the additive, the quantities that can be used, and the way the substance will be identified on labels. ________________________________ refers to substances that are "generally recognized as safe" for consumption and can be added to foods by manufacturers without establishing their safety by rigorous experimental studies. A color additive is any dye, pigment, or substance that can give color when added to a food, drug, or cosmetic or to the human body. Food additives cannot be approved if they cause cancer in humans or animals. This provision of the law is often referred to as the ___________________ ____________________.

Notes

Discovering Nutrition
Second Edition Paul Insel R. Elaine Turner Don Ross

Complementary Nutrition: Functional Foods and Dietary Supplements

Chapter 3

Functional Foods

- Provide health benefits beyond nutrition
- Phytochemicals
  - Antioxidants
    - Neutralize free radicals
    - Reduce heart disease, cancer risk
  - Found in fruits, vegetables, whole grains, legumes, wine

Photos © PhotoDisc

Potential Benefits of Phytochemicals

- Lycopene
  - May reduce risk for cancer, heart disease
- Soy
  - May reduce risk for cancer, heart disease
- Lutein and zeaxanthin
  - May reduce risk for macular degeneration

Notes

Food Additives

- Direct additives
  - Added to foods for specific purpose
- Indirect additives
  - Unintentionally become part of a food

Food Additives

- Purpose of additives
  - Maintain product consistency
  - Improve nutritional value
  - Maintain quality
  - Provide leavening
  - Enhance flavor or color
- Regulated by FDA
- Subject to Delaney Clause

Photos © Corbis Digital Images

Food Additives

- Regulation by FDA
  - Food additives: FDA approval; manufacturer must prove safety
  - Color additives: FDA approval; FDA tests batches for purity
  - Generally Recognized as Safe (GRAS)
  - Prior sanctioned substance
- Subject to Delaney Clause
  - No approval if additive causes cancer

Claims for Functional Foods

- Health claims
- Structure/function claims

Dietary Supplements: Vitamins and Minerals

- Moderate supplementation
  - Increased nutrient needs and/or poor intake
    - Pregnant and breastfeeding women
    - Women with heavy menstrual losses
    - Children
    - Infants
    - People with severe food restrictions
    - Strict vegetarians
    - Elders
  - No more than 150% of DV

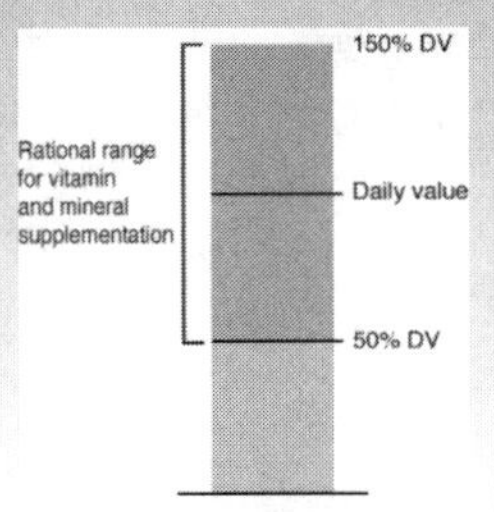

Dietary Supplements: Vitamins and Minerals

- Megadoses
  - Conventional medicine
    - Drug interactions
    - Malabsorption syndromes
    - Treatment of deficiencies
    - Druglike effects
  - Orthomolecular nutrition
    - Proposed for disease prevention
  - Risks: toxicity from large doses

Notes

Notes

Dietary Supplements: Natural Health Products

- Herbal therapy (phytotherapy)
  - Traditional medical practices
  - Little scientific evidence of efficacy, safety
- Helpful herbs: examples
  - St. John's wort
  - Milk thistle
  - Saw palmetto
  - Cranberry

Dietary Supplements: Natural Health Products

- Harmful herbs
  - Potential for drug interactions
  - Examples of products with toxic side effects
    - Yohimbe
    - Ephedra
    - Chaparral
    - Comfrey
- Other types of dietary supplements

Dietary Supplements in the Marketplace

- Regulations
  - Dietary Supplement Health and Education Act
  - FTC: advertising
  - FDA: labeling, content
    - No pre-market approval required
    - Supplement Facts panel
    - Claims

Dietary Supplements in the Marketplace

Serving Size is the manufacturer's suggested serving expressed in the appropriate unit (tablet, capsule, softgel, packet, teaspoonful).

Each Tablet Contains heads the listing of dietary ingredients contained in the supplement.

Each dietary ingredient is followed by the quantity in a serving. For proprietary blends, total weight of the blend is listed, with components listed in descending order by weight.

Dietary ingredients that have no Daily Value are listed below this line.

Botanical supplements must list the part of plant present and its common name (Latin name if common name not listed in *Herbs of Commerce*).

Supplement Facts

Serving Size 1 Tablet

Each Tablet Contains	%DV
Vitamin A 5,000 IU 50% as Beta-Carotene	100%
Vitamin C 90 mg	150%
Vitamin D 400 IU	100%
Vitamin E 45 IU	150%
Thiamin 1.5 mg	100%
Riboflavin 1.7 mg	100%
Niacin 20 mg	100%
Vitamin B_6 2 mg	100%
Folate 400 mcg	100%
Vitamin B_{12} 6 mcg	100%
Calcium 100 mg	10%
Iron 18 mg	100%
Iodine 150 mcg	100%
Magnesium 100 mg	25%
Zinc 15 mg	100%
Ginseng Root (*Panax ginseng*) 25 mg	*
Ginkgo Biloba Leaf (*Ginkgo biloba*) 25 mg	*
Citrus Bioflavonoids Complex 10 mg	*
Lecithin (*Glycine max*) (bean) 10 mg	*
Nickel 5 mcg	*
Silicon 2 mcg	*
Boron 60 mcg	*

* Daily Value (%DV) not established

%DV indicates the percentage of the Daily Value of each nutrient that a serving provides.

An **asterisk** under %DV indicates that a Daily Value is not established for that ingredient.

Dietary Supplements in the Marketplace

- Supplement labels
  - Claims allowed
    - Health claims (approved by FDA)
      - Examples
        - Calcium and osteoporosis
        - Folate and neural tube defects
    - Nutrient content claims

Dietary Supplements in the Marketplace

- Structure/function claims
  - Link substance and effect on the body
  - No approval required
  - Must have "disclaimer" statement on label

Maintains a healthy circulatory system
Maintains a healthy immune system

Helps you relax
Enhances libido
For muscle enhancement

- For common symptoms of PMS
- For hot flashes
- For morning sickness

!

Beware the exclamation point

Notes

Notes

Dietary Supplements in the Marketplace

- Choosing dietary supplements
  - Enough quantity to be effective?
  - How much research has been done?
  - Is it safe?
  - Who is selling the product?
  - Product quality?

DIETARY SUPPLEMENT USP VERIFIED

Dietary Supplements in the Marketplace

- Fraudulent products
  - Secret cure ("breakthrough")
  - Pseudomedical jargon (e.g., "detoxify")
  - Can cure a wide range of diseases
  - Has no side effects, only benefits
  - Backed by "scientific research" you can't find
  - Remember, if it sounds too good to be true…

Complementary and Alternative Medicine (CAM)

- Complementary
  - Practices used in addition to conventional medicine
- Alternative
  - Practices used in place of conventional medicine

NCCAM
National Center for Complementary and Alternative Medicine
National Institutes of Health

Complementary and Alternative Medicine (CAM)

- Nutrition in CAM
  - Vegetarian diets
  - Macrobiotic diet
  - Food restrictions and prescriptions
  - Need for scientific evaluation

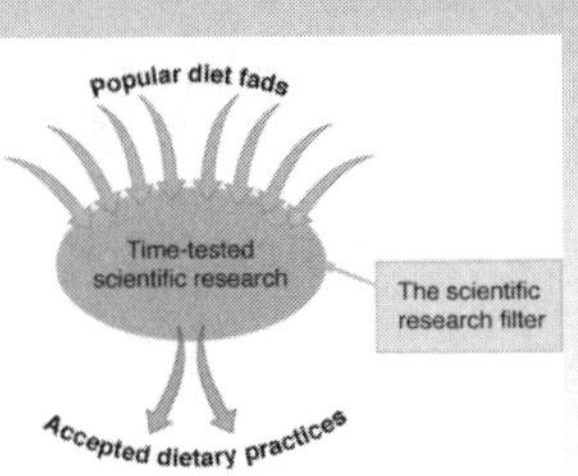

Notes

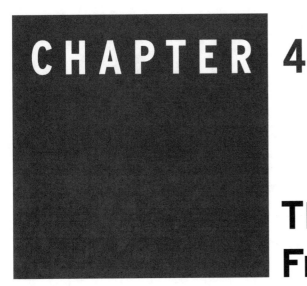

CHAPTER 4

The Human Body: From Food to Fuel

The chapter outline provides you with an organizational guide to the topics and ideas presented in this chapter of the text.

Taste and Smell: The Beginnings of Our Food Experience

The Gastrointestinal Tract
- Organization of the GI Tract

Overview of Digestion: Physical and Chemical Processes
- The Physical Movement and Breaking Up of Food
- The Chemical Breakdown of Food

Overview of Absorption
- The Roads to Nutrient Absorption

Assisting Organs
- Salivary Glands
- Liver
- Gallbladder
- Pancreas

Putting It All Together: Digestion and Absorption
- Mouth
- Stomach
- Small Intestine
- Large Intestine

Circulation of Nutrients
- Vascular System
- Lymphatic System
- Excretion and Elimination

Signaling Systems: Command, Control, and Defense
- Nervous System
- Hormonal System
- Immune System

Influences on Digestion and Absorption
- Psychological Influences
- Chemical Influences
- Bacterial Influences

Nutrition and GI Disorders
- Constipation
- Diarrhea
- Diverticulosis
- Heartburn and Gastroesophageal Reflux Disease
- Irritable Bowel Syndrome
- Colorectal Cancer
- Gas
- Ulcers
- Functional Dyspepsia

◎ Key Terms

Define the following terms.

1. absorption ________________
2. flatulence ________________
3. villi ________________
4. chyme ________________
5. esophagus ________________
6. diverticulitis ________________
7. catalyze ________________
8. diarrhea ________________
9. concentration gradient ________________
10. flatus ________________
11. lumen ________________
12. gastrin ________________
13. segmentation ________________
14. mucosa ________________
15. ulcer ________________
16. bolus ________________
17. passive diffusion ________________
18. intrinsic factor ________________
19. hydrochloric acid ________________
20. sphincters ________________
21. antibodies ________________
22. acrolein ________________
23. pepsinogen ________________
24. hydrolysis ________________
25. ileum ________________
26. digestion ________________
27. emulsifiers ________________
28. irritable bowel syndrome ________________
29. precursor ________________

30. bile ______________________________

31. salivary amylase ______________________________

32. circular muscle ______________________________

33. gallbladder ______________________________

34. enzymes ______________________________

35. mucus ______________________________

36. microvilli ______________________________

37. longitudinal muscle ______________________________

38. pepsin ______________________________

◎ Fill-in-the-Blank

1. The ______________________________ consists of the brain and the spinal cord. It transmits signals that control muscular actions and glandular secretions along the entire GI tract.

2. Chronic pain in the upper abdomen not due to any obvious physical cause is called ______________________________.

3. ______________________________ occurs when small pouches push outward through weak spots in the colon.

4. The movement of substances into or out of cells against a concentration gradient is called ______________________________. This requires energy and involves carrier proteins in the cell membrane.

5. ______________________________ is a fat-splitting enzyme secreted by cells at the base of the tongue.

6. The part of the central nervous system that regulates the automatic responses of the body is the ______________________________.

7. The ______________________________ is a network of nerves located in the gastrointestinal wall.

8. The largest glandular organ in the body, the ______________________________, produces and secretes bile, detoxifies harmful substances, and helps metabolize carbohydrates, lipids, proteins, and micronutrients.

9. ______________________ is a term that refers to the removal of undigested food from the body.

10. The ______________________ is the opening between the esophagus and the stomach that relaxes and opens to allow the bolus to travel into the stomach, and then closes behind it. It also acts as a barrier to prevent the reflux of gastric contents.

11. The middle section of the small intestine (about 120 cm [4 ft] long), lying between the duodenum and ileum, is the ______________________.

12. Infrequent and difficult bowel movements, followed by a sensation of incomplete evacuation, is called ______________________.

13. The ______________________ is a network of veins and arteries through which the blood carries nutrients. It is also called the blood circulatory system.

14. ______________________ is a process by which carrier (transport) proteins in the cell membrane transport substances into or out of cells down a concentration gradient.

15. Recycling of certain compounds between the small intestine and the liver is called ______________________.

16. The ______________________ is the connected series of organs and structures used for digestion of food and absorption of nutrients.

17. The sphincter at the junction of the small and large intestines is the ______________________.

18 Tissue damage to the esophagus due to the reflux of gastric contents is known as ______________________.

19. The ______________________ is a small lymphatic vessel in the interior of each intestinal villus that picks up fat-soluble compounds from intestinal cells.

20. ______________________ is an enzyme in the stomach that primarily breaks down butterfat.

21. The ______________________ secretes enzymes that affect the digestion and absorption of nutrients and that releases hormones, such as insulin, which regulate metabolism as well as the way nutrients are used in the body.

22. The ______________________ is a system of small vessels, ducts, valves, and organized tissue (e.g., lymph nodes) through which lymph moves from its origin in the tissues toward the heart.

23. ______________________________ are the wavelike, rhythmic muscular contractions of the GI tract that propel its contents down the tract.

24. The ______________________________ is a circular muscle that forms the opening between the duodenum and the stomach. It regulates the passage of food into the small intestine.

25. Nonspecific lymphocytes that spontaneously attack and kill cancer cells and cells infected by microorganisms are called ______________________________.

26. The enlarged, muscular, saclike portion of the digestive tract between the esophagus and the small intestine is the ______________________________. It has a capacity of about 1 quart.

27. Large immune system cells that function as patrol cells and engulf and kill foreign invaders are ______________________________.

28. The tube (approximately 3 meters [10 ft] long) where the digestion of protein, fat, and carbohydrate is completed and where the majority of nutrients are absorbed is the ______________________________. It is divided into three parts: the duodenum, the jejunum, and the ileum.

29. ______________________________ are glands in the mouth that release saliva.

30. ______________________________ is a measurement of the hydrogen ion concentration, or acidity, of a solution.

31. The portion of the large intestine extending from the cecum to the rectum is the ______________________________.

32. The ______________________________ is the tube (about 150 cm [5 ft] long) extending from the ileum of the small intestine to the anus. It includes the appendix, cecum, colon, rectum, and anal canal.

33. ______________________________ are substances released at different places in the GI tract to speed the breakdown of ingested carbohydrates, fats, and proteins.

34. ______________________________ are white blood cells that are primarily responsible for immune responses.

35. Burning pain behind the breastbone area caused by acidic stomach contents backing up into the esophagus is called ______________________________.

36. The ______________________________ is the portion of the small intestine closest to the stomach. It is 25 to 30 cm (10 to 12 in.) long and wider than the remainder of the small intestine.

37. Fluid that travels through the lymphatic system, made up of large fat particles and fluid drained from the areas between cells, is called ______________________________.

38. The process of separating and removing waste products of metabolism is ______________________________ ______________________________.

◎ Fill-in-the-Blank Summaries

Putting it All Together: Digestion and Absorption

The digestive process begins in the mouth. Chewing breaks food into smaller pieces, increasing the surface area available to enzymes. Saliva contains the enzyme amylase, which breaks down starch into small sugar molecules. In the mouth, saliva and mucus blend with the food to form a ______________________ ____________________. This ball of chewed food then slides through the esophagus to the stomach. Once in the stomach the ______________________________ keeps the food from sliding back into the esophagus. ______________________________ creates an acidic environment in the stomach that kills many pathogenic bacteria and aids in the digestion of protein. When the chyme is ready to leave the stomach, about 30–40 percent of carbohydrate, 10–20 percent of protein, and less than ____________________ percent of fat have been digested. ______________________________ __ absorption occurs in the stomach. In the small intestine most digestion takes place in the __________ ____________________. Fats do not usually mix with water but this process is facilitated by ____________ ______________________________ once it is released from the gallbladder into the duodenum. Nutrients absorbed through the intestinal lining pass into the interior of the villi. Each villus contains blood vessels and a ____________________. Most minerals with the exception of ______________________, ______________________________, and ______________________________ are absorbed in the small intestine. Undigested material and some liquid move on to the ______________________________ ___, where water and electrolytes are absorbed, leaving waste material to be excreted as feces.

Nutrition and GI Disorders

A diet low in ____________________ and ____________________ and high in ____________________ is the most common cause of constipation. As people age, the colon develops small pouches that bulge outward through weak spots. This condition is known as ______________________________. Eating a diet high in fiber can help prevent this condition. GERD occurs when the lower __________ ____________________ relaxes inappropriately. The esophagus has no protective mucous lining, so acid can quickly damage it. Doctors recommend avoiding foods that can weaken this sphincter such as ______________________________. The cause of IBS remains a mystery. Some foods that are often offenders are __________________ and ______________________. Without treatment, IBS will not progress to a more serious illness. It is likely that a number of physical and psychosocial factors combine to trigger this disorder. After lung cancer, _____________________________ is the most common form of cancer in the United States. Research to date shows that diets high in vegetables and regular physical activity are the most significant factors in reducing risk of this type of cancer. Flatus composition depends largely on ___________________________ intake and the activity of the colon's bacterial population. The major cause of ulcers is _____________________, which creates ulcers by weakening the protective mucous coating around the lining of the stomach.

Notes

Discovering Nutrition
Second Edition Paul Insel R. Elaine Turner Don Ross

The Human Body: From Food to Fuel

Chapter 4

The Gastrointestinal Tract

- Organization
  - Mouth ← anus
  - Accessory organs
    - Salivary glands, liver, pancreas, gallbladder

The Gastrointestinal Tract

- Functions
  - Ingestion
  - Transport
  - Secretion
  - Digestion
  - Absorption
  - Elimination

Overview of Digestion

- Physical movement
  - Peristalsis
  - Segmentation
- Chemical breakdown
  - Enzymes
  - Other secretions

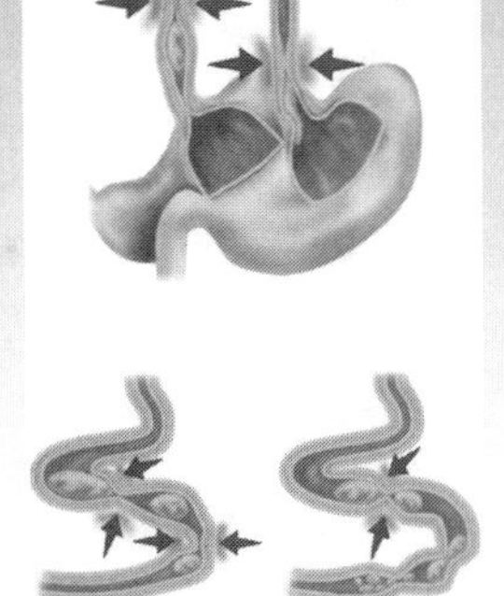

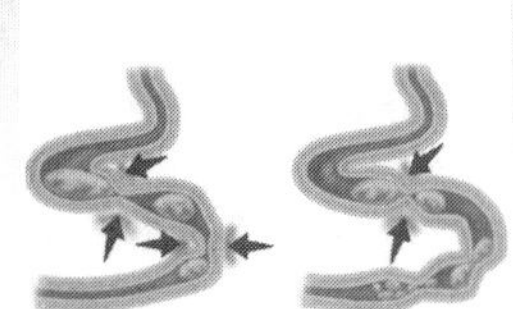

Overview of Absorption

- Absorptive mechanisms
  - Passive diffusion
  - Facilitated diffusion
  - Active transport

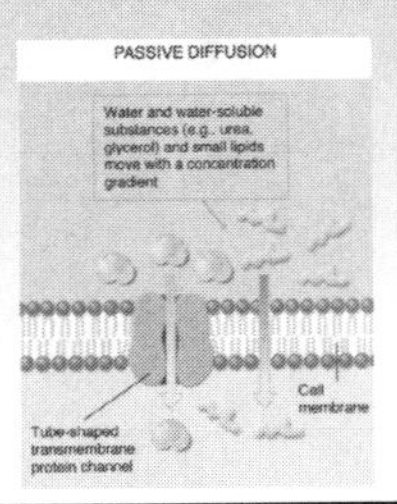

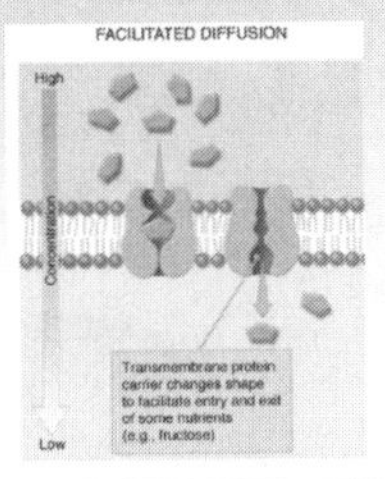

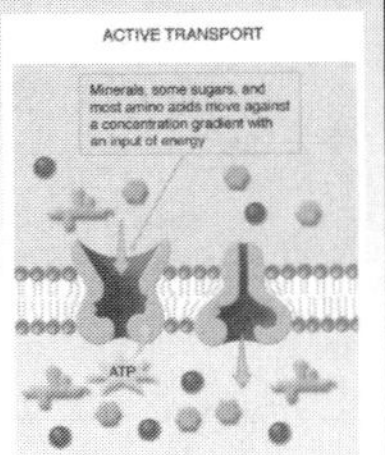

Assisting Organs

- Salivary glands
  - Moisten food
  - Supply enzymes
- Liver
  - Produces bile
- Gallbladder
  - Stores and secretes bile
- Pancreas
  - Secretes bicarbonate
  - Secretes enzymes

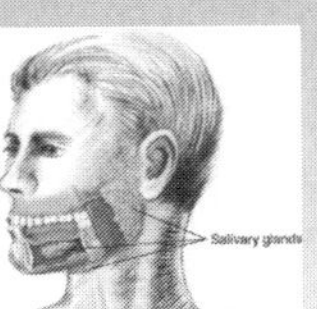

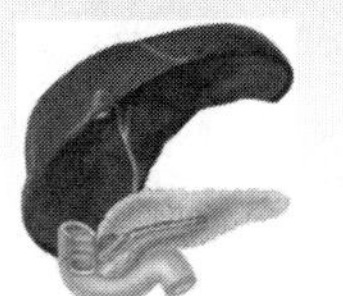

Notes

Notes

Putting It All Together: Digestion and Absorption

- Mouth
  - Enzymes
    - Salivary amylase acts on starch
    - Lingual lipase acts on fat
  - Saliva
    - Moistens food for swallowing
- Esophagus
  - Transports food to stomach
  - Esophageal sphincter

Putting It All Together: Digestion and Absorption

- Stomach
  - Hydrochloric acid
    - Prepares protein for digestion
    - Activates enzymes
  - Pepsin
    - Begins protein digestion
  - Gastric lipase
    - Some fat digestion
  - Gastrin (hormone)
    - Stimulates gastric secretion and movement
  - Intrinsic factor
    - Needed for absorption of vitamin B_{12}

Putting It All Together: Digestion and Absorption

- Small intestine
  - Sections of small intestine
    - Duodenum, jejunum, ileum
  - Digestion
    - Bicarbonate neutralizes stomach acid
    - Pancreatic and intestinal enzymes
      - Carbohydrates
      - Fat
      - Protein

Putting It All Together: Digestion and Absorption

- Small intestine
  - Absorption
    - Folds, villi, and microvilli expand absorptive surface
    - Most nutrients absorbed here
    - Fat-soluble nutrients go into lymph
    - Other nutrients go into blood

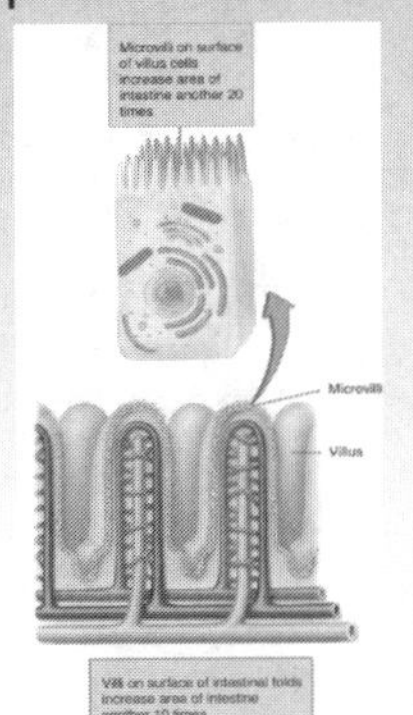

Putting It All Together: Digestion and Absorption

- Large intestine
  - Digestion
    - Nutrient digestion already complete
    - Some digestion of fiber by bacteria
  - Absorption
    - Water
    - Sodium, potassium, chloride
    - Vitamin K (produced by bacteria)
  - Elimination

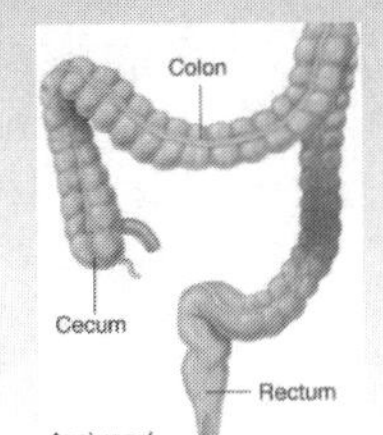

Circulation of Nutrients

- Vascular system
  - Veins and arteries
  - Carries oxygen and nutrients to tissues
  - Removes wastes
- Lymphatic system
  - Vessels that drain lymph

Notes

Notes

Circulation of Nutrients

- Excretion and elimination
  - Lungs
    - Excrete water and carbon dioxide
  - Kidneys filter blood
    - Excrete waste, maintain water and ion balance

Signaling Systems: Command, Control, Defense

- Nervous system
  - Regulates GI activity
    - Local system of nerves
    - Central nervous system
- Hormonal system
  - Increases or decreases GI activity

Signaling Systems: Command, Control, Defense

- Immune system
  - Identifies and attacks foreign invaders
  - Role of GI tract
    - Barrier
    - Location of lymphoid tissue

Influences on Digestion and Absorption

- Chemical influences
- Bacterial influences

Nutrition and GI Disorders

- Constipation
  - Hard, dry, infrequent stools
  - Reduced by high fiber, fluid intake, exercise
- Diarrhea
  - Loose, watery, frequent stools
  - Symptom of diseases/infections
  - Can cause dehydration

Nutrition and GI Disorders

- Diverticulosis
  - Pouches along colon
  - High-fiber diet reduces formation
- Heartburn and GERD
  - Reduced by smaller meals, less fat
- Irritable bowel syndrome

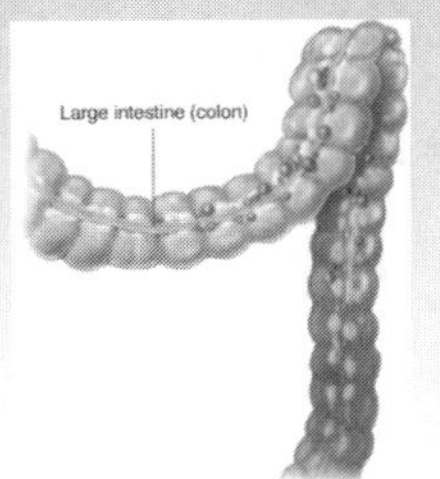

Notes

Notes

Nutrition and GI Disorders

- Colorectal cancer
  - Antioxidants may reduce risk
- Gas
- Ulcers
  - Bacterial cause
- Functional dyspepsia

Nutrition and GI Disorders

- Gastroesophageal reflux disease (GERD)
  - Reduced by smaller meals, less fat
- Irritable bowel syndrome (IBS)
- Colon cancer
  - Antioxidants may reduce risk
- Gas
- Ulcers
  - Bacterial cause
- Functional dyspepsia

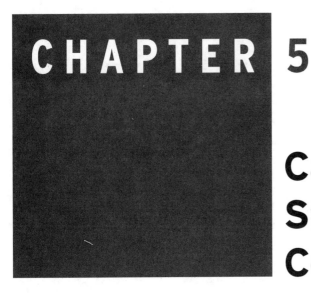

CHAPTER 5

Carbohydrates: Simple Sugars and Complex Chains

The chapter outline provides you with an organizational guide to the topics and ideas presented in this chapter of the text.

◎ Key Terms

Define the following terms.

1. **acesulfame K** ______________________________

2. **total fiber** ______________________________

3. **insulin resistance** ______________________________

4. **glycemic index** ______________________________

5. pectins _____

6. husk _____

7. endosperm _____

8. germ _____

9. fasting hypoglycemia _____

10. complex carbohydrates _____

11. functional fiber _____

12. alpha bonds _____

13. epinephrine _____

14. fructose _____

15. dietary fiber _____

16. aspartame _____

17. amylase _____

18. lignins _____

19. trehalose _____

20. ketosis _____

21. neotame _____

22. nutritive sweeteners _____

23. dental caries _____

24. galactose _____

25. glucose _____

26. resistant starch _____

27. lactose _____

28. pancreatic amylase _____

29. maltose _____

30. sucralose _____

31. starch _____

32. saccharin _____

◎ Fill-in-the-Blank

1. _____ are a group of large polysaccharides in dietary fiber that are fermented more easily than cellulose.

2. ______________________________ are branched polysaccharide chains of glucose found in barley and oats. They help to lower blood cholesterol levels.

3. A chronic disease in which uptake of blood glucose by body cells is impaired, resulting in high glucose levels in the blood and urine, is ______________.

4. Sugars composed of a single sugar molecule (a monosaccharide) or two joined sugar molecules (a disaccharide) are ______________________.

5. ______________________________ occurs when the body's immune system attacks the pancreas, causing its cells to lose the ability to make insulin; ______________________________ occurs when target cells (e.g., fat and muscle cells) lose the ability to respond normally to insulin.

6. Dietary fibers that contain galactose and other monosaccharides and that are found between plant cell walls are ______________________.

7. An abnormally high concentration of glucose in the blood is called ______________________, while an abnormally low concentration of glucose in the blood is ______________________.

8. The layers of protective coating around the grain kernel that are rich in dietary fiber and nutrients are called the ______________________.

9. ______________________________ is a condition that results in high blood glucose levels during pregnancy.

10. ______________________________ is an artificial sweetener derived from lactose that has the same sweetness as sucrose with only half the calories.

11. ______________________________ are chemical bonds linking monosaccharides, which sometimes cannot be broken by human intestinal enzymes. Lactose contains digestible ones, and cellulose contains nondigestible ones.

12. A branched-chain polysaccharide in food composed of glucose units is ______________________.

13. Produced by the pancreas, ______________________ promotes the breakdown of liver glycogen to glucose, and so increases blood glucose levels.

14. ______________________________ are carbohydrates composed of two monosaccharide units chemically linked. They include sucrose (common table sugar), lactose (milk sugar), and maltose.

15. The dried husk of the psyllium seed is ________________________________.

16. ____ are single sugar units. The common kinds are glucose, fructose, and galactose.

17. ____ is a very large, highly branched polysaccharide composed of multiple glucose units. Sometimes called animal starch, it is the primary storage form of glucose in animals.

18. Molecules formed from fat when cells do not have enough available carbohydrate to break down fat completely are called ____________________________________.

19. ____ is a long-chain structural polysaccharide of slightly modified glucose. Found in the hard exterior skeletons of insects, crustaceans, and other invertebrates, it also occurs in the cell walls of fungi. A polysaccharide derived from this is ____________ __________________________.

20. ____ is an inherited disorder in which the enzyme that metabolizes phenylalanine is missing.

21. Substances that impart sweetness to foods but supply little or no energy to the body are called ________ ____.

22. Short carbohydrate chains composed of 3 to 10 sugar molecules are ____________________________ __________________.

23. Produced by the pancreas, ____ stimulates the uptake of blood glucose into cells, the formation of glycogen in the liver, and various other processes.

24. ____ are gel-forming dietary fibers containing galactose, mannose, and other monosaccharides; they are found in seaweed.

25. ____ is a disaccharide composed of glucose and fructose; it is also known as table sugar.

26. ____ is a dietary supplement, not approved for use as a sweetener, that is extracted and refined from Stevia rebaudiana leaves.

27. ____ is a type of hypoglycemia that occurs about one hour after eating carbohydrate-rich food. The body overreacts and produces too much insulin in response to food, rapidly decreasing blood glucose levels.

28. ____ is a condition in which blood glucose levels are higher than normal but not high enough to warrant a diagnosis of diabetes.

29. ______________________________ are compounds formed from monosaccharides and are commonly used as nutritive sweeteners; they are also called polyols.

30. Long carbohydrate chains composed of more than 10 sugar molecules are called ______________ ______________. They can be straight or branched.

31. ______________________________ are substances composed of monosaccharides and disaccharides that have been extracted and processed from other foods.

◎ Fill-in-the-Blank Summaries

What Are Carbohydrates?

Carbohydrates are organic compounds that contain carbon, oxygen, and hydrogen. The two main types of sugars are monosaccharides and disaccharides. Glucose, ______________, and fructose are the three most common ______________. Disaccharides are created when ______________ ______ monosaccharides are joined. ______________ is the most abundant simple carbohydrate unit in nature. It makes up at least one of the two sugar molecules in every ______________. ______________, also known as levulose, tastes the sweetest of all sugars. ______________ ______________ is usually chemically bonded to glucose to form lactose.

When a food label lists sugar as an ingredient the term refers to ______________. Human milk tastes sweeter than cow's milk because it has a higher concentration of lactose. When digestive enzymes break down starch in the mouth, a sweet taste is sensed. This sweet taste can be attributed to ______________ ______________.

Complex Carbohydrates

Oligosaccharides are ______________ carbohydrate chains of ______ to ______ sugar molecules. Long carbohydrate chains are known as ______________, and are composed of more than ______________ sugar molecules. Starches are polysaccharides. There are two main forms of starch in plants. Amylose is made of long, straight chains of glucose molecules; amylopectin is made of branched chains of glucose molecules.

In human cells, glycogen can be broken down rapidly into single glucose molecules. ______________ ______________ and the liver are the two main sites of glycogen storage. The liver uses glycogen to regulate blood glucose levels.

There are many types of dietary fiber. The ______________________________ in fruit gives fruit its body; when it breaks down fruit becomes mushy.

______________________________ fibers dissolve in water, while ______________________________ fibers do not. Wheat bran and most whole grain cereals are rich in insoluble fibers. When fiber intake increases so should water intake to avoid excess intestinal gas and bloating.

Carbohydrates in the Body

Lately Danny has not felt like himself. Soon after his 15th birthday he began feeling thirsty all of the time, urinating frequently, and experiencing nausea. Due to Danny's age and symptoms, it is likely that he has developed ______________________________. ______________________________ is the hallmark of Danny's ailment. It is called the disease of "starvation in the midst of plenty" because although blood glucose levels are high the carbohydrate cannot ______________________________.

Type 2 diabetes is the most common form of diabetes. The risk of developing this type of diabetes increases as fat storage increases in the ______________________________. Sometimes this type of diabetes can be managed by only ______________________________.

______________________________ occurs when blood glucose levels are too low. A person with diabetes develops this in response to ______________________________. If the body produces too much insulin in response to food, the result is reactive hypoglycemia.

Notes

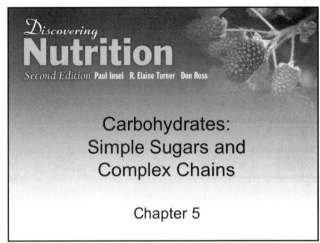

Carbohydrates:
Simple Sugars and
Complex Chains

Chapter 5

Carbohydrates

- Sugars, starches, fibers
- Major food sources: plants
  - Formed during photosynthesis

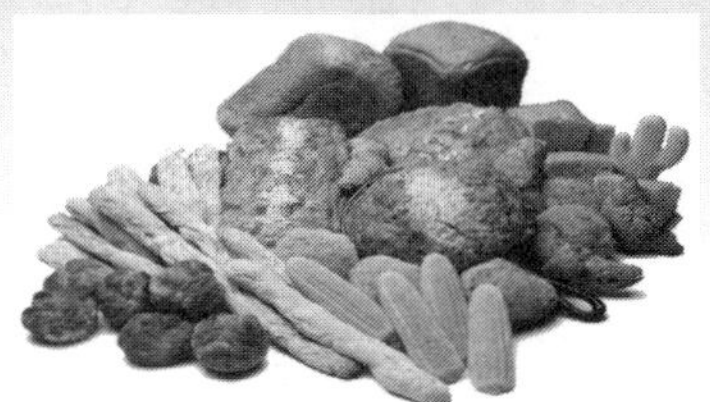

Photo © PhotoDisc

Monosaccharides: The Single Sugars

- Monosaccharides: single sugar units
  - Glucose
    - Found in fruits, vegetables, honey
    - "blood sugar"—used for energy
  - Fructose
    - "Fruit sugar"
    - Found in fruits, honey, corn syrup
  - Galactose
    - Found as part of lactose in milk

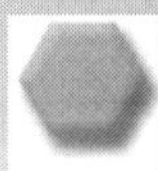

Glucose

Fructose

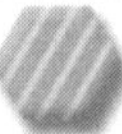

Galactose

Notes

Disaccharides: The Double Sugars

- Disaccharides: two linked sugar units
  - Sucrose: glucose + fructose
    - "Table sugar"
    - Made from sugar cane and sugar beets
  - Lactose: glucose + galactose
    - "Milk sugar"
    - Found in milk and dairy products
  - Maltose: glucose + glucose
    - Found in germinating cereal grains
    - Product of starch breakdown

Sucrose

Lactose

Maltose

Complex Carbohydrates

- Starch
  - Long chains of glucose units
    - Amylose—straight chains
    - Amylopectin—branched chains
  - Found in grains, vegetables, legumes
- Glycogen
  - Highly branched chains of glucose units
  - Body's storage form of carbohydrate

Starch (amylose)

Glycogen

Complex Carbohydrates

- Fiber
  - Indigestible chains of monosaccharides
  - Dietary fiber: found in plants
    - Fruits, vegetables, grains, legumes
  - Functional fiber: isolated and added to foods

Complex Carbohydrates

- Types of fiber
  - Oligosaccharides: short chains of monosaccharides
    - Raffinose, stachyose
  - Cellulose
  - Hemicellulose
  - Pectins
  - Gums and cilages
  - Lignins
  - Beta-glucans
  - Chitin and chitosan

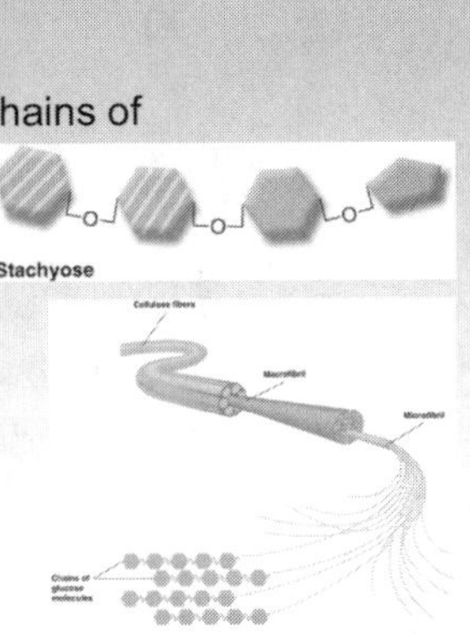

Carbohydrate Digestion and Absorption

- Mouth
  - Salivary amylase begins digestion of starch
- Small intestine
  - Pancreatic amylase completes starch digestion
  - Brush border enzymes digest disaccharides

Carbohydrate Digestion and Absorption

- End products of carbohydrate digestion
  - Glucose, fructose, galactose
  - Absorbed into bloodstream
- Fibers are not digested; excreted in feces

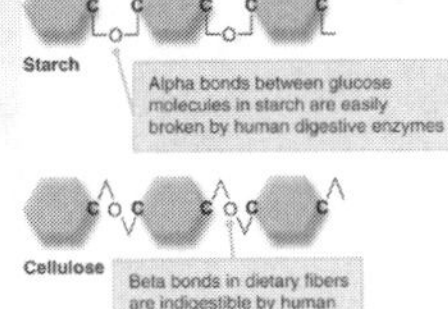

Notes

Notes

Carbohydrates in Action

- Functions of carbohydrates
  - Energy source
    - Glucose is the body's main fuel
  - Excess glucose is stored as glycogen
    - Stored in liver and muscle
  - Adequate glucose
    - Spares protein
    - Prevents ketosis

Glycogen

Carbohydrates in Action: Regulating Blood Glucose

High blood glucose
Insulin released
Insulin stimulates cells to take up glucose from the blood
Pancreas
Blood glucose
Insulin stimulates liver and muscle cells to store glucose as glycogen
(a)

Low blood glucose
Glucagon released
Glucagon stimulates liver cells to break down glycogen to glucose
Glucagon stimulates liver cells to make glucose from amino acids
(b)

Carbohydrates in Action

- Diabetes mellitus
  - Persistent high blood glucose levels
  - Type 1 diabetes: lack of insulin production
  - Type 2 diabetes: cells are resistant to insulin
  - Gestational diabetes: occurs during pregnancy

Carbohydrates in Action

- Risk factors for type 2 diabetes
  - Age
  - Overweight
  - Family history
  - Lack of exercise
  - Ethnicity

Carbohydrates in Your Diet

- Recommended carbohydrate intake
  - RDA = 130 grams per day
  - AMDR = 45–65% of calories
  - Daily Value (for 2,000 kcal) = 300 grams
  - *Dietary Guidelines*
    - Choose/prepare foods with little added sugar
    - Choose fiber-rich fruits, vegetables, whole grains often

Carbohydrates in Your Diet

- Choosing carbohydrates wisely
  - Whole grains
  - Legumes
  - Vegetables
  - Fruit

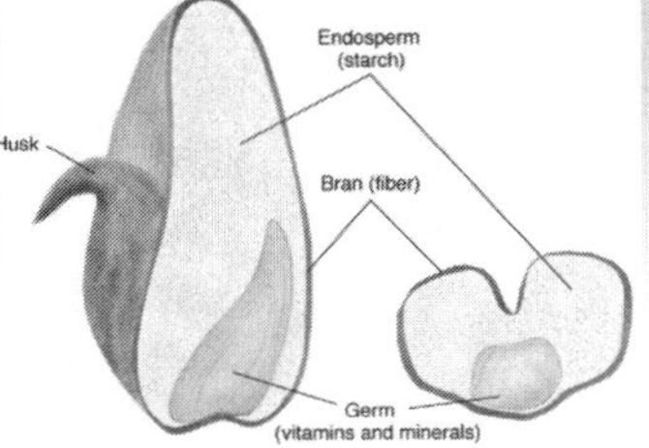

Notes

Notes

Carbohydrates in Your Diet

- Moderating sugar intake
  - Use less added sugar
  - Limit soft drinks, sugary cereals, candy
  - Choose fresh fruits or those canned in water or juice

Photo © CSquared Studios/PhotoDisc

Carbohydrates in Your Diet

- Nutritive sweeteners
  - Natural vs. refined
  - Sugar alcohols
- Non-nutritive sweeteners
  - Saccharin
  - Aspartame
  - Acesulfame K
  - Sucralose

Relative sweetness (sucrose = 1)
300
100
30
10
3
1
0.3
Sucrose
Lactose
Maltose
Glucose
Fructose
Sorbitol
Aspartame
Saccharin
Acesulfame
Key Sugar alcohol
Refined sweeteners
Artificial sweetners

Carbohydrates and Health

- Sugar
  - High sugar intake may be low in nutrients
  - High sugar intake promotes tooth decay

Carbohydrates and Health

- Fiber
  - Improves weight control
  - Better control of blood glucose
  - Reduced risk of heart disease
  - Healthier gastrointestinal functioning

Notes

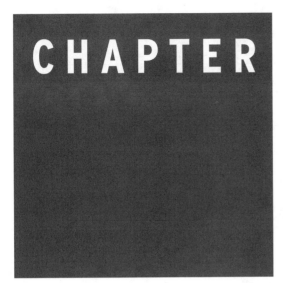

CHAPTER 6

Lipids: Not Just Fat

The chapter outline provides you with an organizational guide to the topics and ideas presented in this chapter of the text.

◎ Key Terms

Define the following terms.

1. **adipocytes** ______________________________

2. **squalene** ______________________________

3. **diglyceride** ______________________________

4. subcutaneous fat ______________________________

5. cholesterol______________________________

6. visceral fat______________________________

7. metabolic syndrome______________________________

8. hypercholesterolemia ______________________________

9. chain length______________________________

10. hydrogenation______________________________

11. lanugo ______________________________

12. therapeutic lifestyle changes (TLC) ______________________________

13. phytosterols______________________________

14. *omega*-3 fatty acid ______________________________

15. micelles ______________________________

16. adipose tissue ______________________________

17. eicosanoids ______________________________

18. very-low-density lipoproteins (VLDL) ______________________________

19. *omega*-6 fatty acid ______________________________

20. monounsaturated fatty acid ______________________________

21. atherosclerosis ______________________________

22. intermediate-density lipoproteins (IDL) ______________________________

23. sterols ______________________________

24. oxidation______________________________

25. phosphate group ______________________________

26. polyunsaturated fatty acid______________________________

27. obesity ______________________________

◎ Fill-in-the-Blank

1. The major enzyme responsible for the breakdown of lipoproteins and triglycerides in the blood is

______________________________.

2. ______________________________ is an essential *omega*-3 fatty acid that contains 18 carbon atoms and 3 carbon–carbon double bonds.

3. A term for diseases in which abnormal cells divide without control is ______________________________.

These cells can invade nearby tissues and can spread through the bloodstream and lymphatic system to other parts of the body.

4. A ______________________________ is an unsaturated fatty acid with a bent carbon chain. Most naturally occurring unsaturated fatty acids are these.

5. ______________________________ is the backbone of mono-, di-, and triglycerides; alone, it is a thick, smooth liquid.

6. ______________________________ are fatty acids that the body needs but cannot synthesize and must obtain from the diet.

7. ______________________________ is a fat replacer made from a sucrose backbone with six to eight fatty acids attached. The fatty acid arrangement prevents breakdown by the digestive enzyme lipase, so the fatty acids are not absorbed. It can withstand heat and is stable at frying temperatures. Trade name is Olean.

8. ______________________________ are compounds containing a long hydrocarbon chain with a carboxyl group (–COOH) at one end and a methyl group ($–CH_3$) at the other end.

9. A fatty acid in which the carbon chain contains one or more double bonds is an ______________________________.

10. ______________________________ are compounds that consist of a glycerol molecule bonded to two fatty acid molecules and phosphate group with a nitrogen-containing component. They have both water-soluble and fat-soluble regions, which make them good emulsifiers.

11. The blood lipoproteins that contain high levels of protein and low levels of triglycerides are called ______________________________. Synthesized primarily in the liver and small intestine, these pick up cholesterol released from dying cells and other sources and transfers it to other lipoproteins. They are sometimes called “good cholesterol.”

12. ______________________________ is a protein released by the body in response to acute injury, infection, or other inflammatory stimuli. It is associated with future cardiovascular events.

13. A molecule of glycerol combined with one fatty acid is a ____________________.

14. A general term for all disorders affecting the heart and blood vessels is ______________________________.

15. ______________________________ are the cholesterol-rich lipoproteins that result from the breakdown and removal of triglycerides from intermediate-density lipoprotein. Sometimes called "bad cholesterol."

16. ______________________________ is a substance that consists of an LDL part plus a protein (apoprotein a) whose exact function is currently unknown.

17. A fatty acid completely filled by hydrogen, with all carbons in the chain linked by single bonds is a ______________________________.

18. ______________________________ is an essential *omega*-6 fatty acid that contains 18 carbon atoms and 2 carbon–carbon double bonds (18:2); it is a thin liquid at room temperature.

19. ______________________________ are compounds that imitate the functional and sensory properties of fats, but contain less available energy than fats.

20. ______________________________ is a nitrogen-containing compound that is part of phosphatidylcholine, a phospholipid. It also is part of the neurotransmitter acetylcholine. The body can synthesize it from the amino acid methionine.

21. In the body, ______________________________ is a phospholipid with the nitrogen-containing component choline. In foods, it is a blend of phospholipids with different nitrogen-containing components.

22. A ______________________________ is an unsaturated fatty acid with a straighter chain than a *cis* fatty acid, usually as a result of hydrogenation; it is more solid than a *cis* fatty acid.

23. A ______________________________ is a large lipoprotein formed in intestinal cells following the absorption of dietary fats. It has a central core of triglycerides and cholesterol surrounded by phospholipids and proteins.

24. ______________________________ are fatty acids that your body can make when they are needed. It is not necessary to consume them in the diet.

25. A ______________________________ is a complex that transports lipids in the lymph and blood. It consists of a central core of triglycerides and cholesterol surrounded by a shell composed of proteins, cholesterol, and phospholipids. The various types differ in size, composition, and density.

◎ Fill-in-the-Blank Summaries

Fatty Acids Are Key Building Blocks

Lipids are a broad range of molecules that dissolve easily in organic solvents, but are much less soluble in ______________________________. They are generally hydrophobic and lipophilic. The three main types of lipids are triglycerides, phospholipids, and sterols. ______________________________ are the largest category of lipids and are stored in the body in ______________________________. ______________________________ are major building blocks of cell membranes. They keep fats suspended in watery fluids. The most famous sterol, cholesterol, is manufactured in the body and is a precursor to the synthesis of sex hormones, ______________________________, and vitamin D. Lipids share many of the same functional properties and transport mechanisms.

______________________________ are common components of triglycerides and phospholipids. There are many types of these substances, which are basically chains of ______________________________ atoms with a carboxyl group on one end and a methyl group at the other end. Short chain fatty acids have less than ______________________________ carbons; medium chains have 6–10; and long chains have ______________________________ or more. The water-soluble property of shorter fatty acids affects their absorption.

A triglyceride is made of ______________________________ fatty acids attached to a glycerol molecule. Triglycerides are esters which form when a hydrogen and an oxygen from the carboxyl group combine with a hydrogen atom from the alcohol's hydroxyl group. A molecule of water is produced which makes this a ______________________________ reaction.

Lipids in the Body and the Diet

Lipoprotein carriers transport lipids through the bloodstream. Chylomicrons are formed in the ______________________________. They eventually reach the bloodstream through the ______________________________ in the neck. As they travel through the bloodstream they gradually give up triglycerides to capillary walls. Lipoprotein lipase breaks them down. After ______________________________ hours little is left of the chylomicron except cholesterol-rich remnants.

HDLs are scavenger lipoproteins, picking up excess ______________________________ released by dying cells and arterial plaques. These plaques are created by LDL degrading over a long period of time. ______________________________ that have embedded themselves in arterial walls damaged by smoking or diabetes have scavenger receptors which bind to LDL and cause it to release its cholesterol. If HDL levels are low there is an increased risk for atherosclerotic heart disease.

The Daily Value on food labels recommends consuming ______________ grams of fat based on a 2000 kcalorie diet. To fulfill the need for *omega*-6 fatty acids, linoleic acid should provide 2% of our calories.

When protein is used as part of a fat substitute, the product cannot be used in cooking because high temperatures cause denaturation. Many products use carbohydrates as fat replacements and bind ____ to further dilute calories. Olestra is a very controversial fat substitute. Because olestra is not absorbed, it may cause symptoms of fat malabsorption such as ____.

Notes

Discovering Nutrition

Second Edition Paul Insel R. Elaine Turner Don Ross

Lipids: Not Just Fat

Chapter 6

Lipids

- Triglycerides (fats and oils)
- Phospholipids
- Cholesterol

Photo © PhotoDisc

Fatty Acids Are Key Building Blocks

Short-chain fatty acid (2-4 carbons)

Butyric C4:0

Medium-chain fatty acid (6-10 carbons)

Caprylic C8:0

Long-chain fatty acid (12 or more carbons)

Palmitic C16:0

- Chain length
  - 4 to 24 carbons

Notes

Fatty Acids Are Key Building Blocks

- Saturation
  - Saturated fatty acid
    - All single bonds between carbons
  - Monounsaturated fatty acid
    - One carbon–carbon double bond
  - Polyunsaturated fatty acid
    - More than one carbon–carbon double bond

Fatty Acids Are Key Building Blocks

- *Cis* vs. *trans*
  - *Cis* fatty acids
    - Occur naturally
    - Chain is bent
  - *Trans* fatty acids
    - Produced by hydrogenation
    - Chain is straighter

Cis form (bent)

Trans form (straighter)

Fatty Acids Are Key Building Blocks

- Essential and nonessential fatty acids
  - Essential fatty acids
    - Can't be made in the body
    - Linoleic acid and *alpha*-linolenic acid
    - Used to make eicosanoids "local hormones"

Your body cannot form C=C double bonds **before** the 9th carbon

Your body can form C=C double bonds **after** the 9th carbon

Fatty acids with double bonds before the 9th carbon are ESSENTIAL

Linolenic acid

Linoleic acid

Fatty Acids Are Key Building Blocks

- Essential and nonessential fatty acids
  - Nonessential fatty acids
    - Can be made in the body

Triglycerides

- Structure
  - Glycerol + three fatty acids
- Functions
  - Energy source
    - 9 kcal/g
    - Form of stored energy in adipose tissue
  - Insulation and protection
  - Carrier of fat-soluble vitamins
  - Sensory qualities in food

Triglycerides in Food

- Sources of *omega*-3 fatty acids
  - Soybean, canola, walnut, flaxseed oils
  - Salmon, tuna, mackerel
- Sources of *omega*-6 fatty acids
  - Vegetable oils

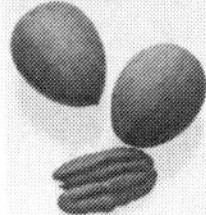
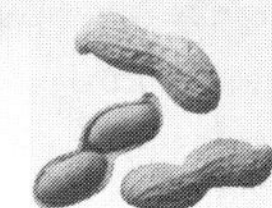
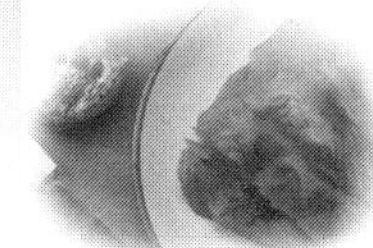

Notes

Notes

Phospholipids

- Structure
  - Glycerol + two fatty acids + phosphate group
- Functions
  - Component of cell membranes
  - Lipid transport as part of lipoproteins
  - Emulsifiers
- Food sources
  - Egg yolks, liver, soybeans, peanuts

Sterols: Cholesterol

- Functions
  - Component of cell membranes
  - Precursor to other substances
    - Sterol hormones
    - Vitamin D
    - Bile acids
- Synthesis
  - Made in the liver
- Food sources
  - Found only in animal foods

Cholesterol

Lipid Digestion and Absorption

- Mouth and stomach
  - Minimal digestion of triglycerides
- Small intestine
  - Emulsified by phospholipids
  - Digested by pancreatic lipase
  - Absorbed into intestinal cells
    - Formed into chylomicrons and moved into lymphatic system

Lipids in the Body

- Lipoproteins carry lipids around the body
  - Chylomicrons
    - Deliver dietary lipids from intestines to cells and liver

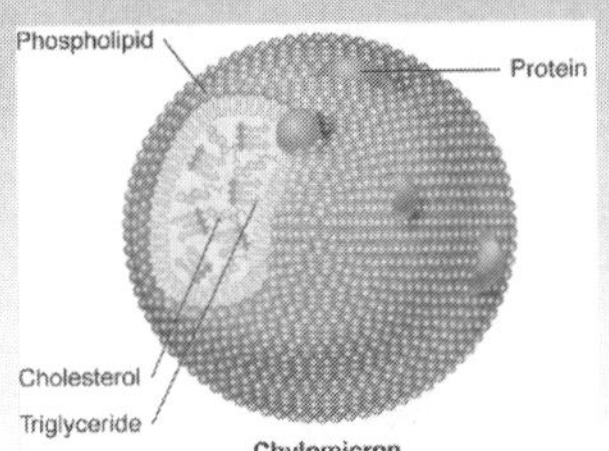

Lipids in the Body

- Very-low-density lipoproteins (VLDL)
  - Deliver triglycerides to cells
- Low-density lipoproteins (LDL)
  - Deliver cholesterol to cells
- High-density lipoproteins (HDL)
  - Pick up cholesterol for removal or recycling

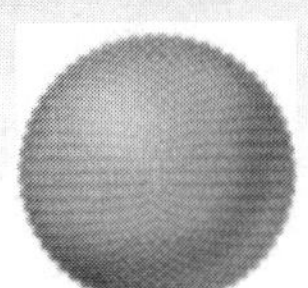

Lipids in the Diet

- Recommended intake
  - Reduce saturated and *trans* fat intake
  - Total fat: 20–35% of calories
  - Need approximately 2% of kilocalories as essential fatty acids
  - Improve balance of *omega*-3 and *omega*-6 fatty acids

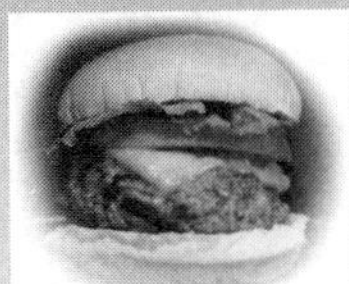

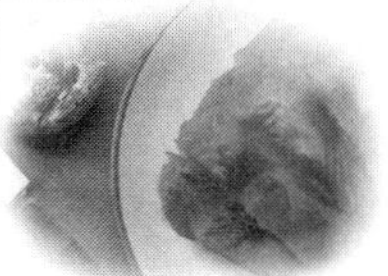

Notes

Notes

Lipids in the Diet

- Fat replacers
  - Different types of composition
  - Olestra
    - Sucrose + fatty acids
    - Indigestible—provides no calories
    - Reduces absorption of fat-soluble vitamins

Fatty acid
Fatty acid
Fatty acid
Fatty acid
Fatty acid
Fatty acid
Fatty acid
Fatty acid

Lipids and Health

- Obesity
  - High-fat diets promote weight gain
- Heart disease
  - Major risk factors
    - High blood cholesterol
      - High LDL and low HDL
    - Smoking
    - High blood pressure

Lipids and Health

- Reducing heart disease risk
  - Lifestyle
    - Stop smoking
    - Increase exercise
    - Manage weight
    - Manage blood pressure

Lipids and Health

- Reducing heart disease risk
  - Diet
    - Reduce saturated fat, cholesterol, total fat
    - Increase antioxidants
    - Increase B vitamins
    - Increase *omega*-3 fatty acids
    - Increase dietary fiber
    - Other factors

Lipids and Health

- Metabolic syndrome
  - Cluster of at least three symptoms
    - Excess abdominal fat
    - High blood glucose
    - High serum triglycerides
    - Low HDL cholesterol
    - High blood pressure

Lipids and Health

- Cancer
  - Stages of development
    - Initiation
    - Promotion
    - Progression
  - Role of diet
    - Factors that promote or protect

Notes

Notes

Lipids and Health

- Cancer
  - Reducing cancer risk
    - Eat a variety of healthful foods; plant sources
    - Be more physically active
    - Maintain a healthful weight
    - Limit alcohol consumption

CHAPTER 7

Proteins and Amino Acids: Function Follows Form

The chapter outline provides you with an organizational guide to the topics and ideas presented in this chapter of the text.

Why Is Protein Important?

Amino Acids Are the Building Blocks of Proteins
- Amino Acids Are Identified by Their Side Groups
- Protein Structure: Unique Three-Dimensional Shapes and Functions
- Protein Denaturation: Destabilizing a Protein's Shape

Functions of Body Proteins
- Structural and Mechanical Functions
- Immune Function
- Enzymes
- Hormones
- Acid-Base Balance
- Transport Functions
- Fluid Balance
- Source of Energy and Glucose

Protein Digestion and Absorption
- Protein Digestion
- Amino Acid and Peptide Absorption
- Undigested Protein

Proteins in the Body
- Protein Synthesis
- The Amino Acid Pool and Protein Turnover
- Synthesis of Nonprotein Molecules
- Protein and Nitrogen Excretion
- Nitrogen Balance

Proteins in the Diet
- Recommended Intakes of Protein
- Protein Consumption in the United States
- Protein Quality
- Evaluating Protein Quality
- Proteins and Amino Acids as Additives and Supplements

The Pros and Cons of Vegetarian Eating
- Why People Become Vegetarians
- Types of Vegetarians
- Health Benefits of Vegetarian Diets
- Health Risks of Vegetarian Diets
- Dietary Recommendations for Vegetarians

The Health Effects of Too Little or Too Much Protein
- Protein-Energy Malnutrition
- Excess Dietary Protein

◎ Key Terms

Define the following terms.

1. **amino acid pool** ______________________________

2. **incomplete proteins** ______________________________

3. **tripeptide** ______________________________

4. **wasting** ______________________________

5. **deamination** ______________________________

6. **marasmus** ______________________________

7. **acidosis** ______________________________

8. **alkalosis** ______________________________

9. **edema** ______________________________

10. **buffers** ______________________________

11. **complete proteins** ______________________________

12. **proenzymes** ______________________________

13. **dipeptide** ______________________________

14. **complementary proteins** ______________________________

15. **kwashiorkor** ______________________________

16. **protein digestibility-corrected amino acid score (PDCAAS)** ______________________________

17. **nitrogen equilibrium** ______________________________

18. **antibodies** ______________________________

19. **proteases** ______________________________

20. **polypeptide** ______________________________

21. **nitrogen balance** ______________________________

22. **immune response** ______________________________

23. **oligopeptide** ______________________________

24. **intravascular fluid** ______________________________

◎ Fill-in-the-Blank

1. Proteins that use energy and convert it into some form of mechanical work are ____________________ ____________________. They are active in processes such as cell division, muscle contraction, and sperm movement.

2. ______________________________ is a disease that involves an inability to digest gluten, a protein found in wheat, rye, oats, and barley. If untreated, it causes flattening of the villi in the intestine, leading to severe malabsorption of nutrients. Symptoms include diarrhea, fatty stools, swollen belly, and extreme fatigue.

3. The bond between two amino acids formed when a carboxyl (–COOH) group of one amino acid joins an amino (–NH_2) group of another amino acid, releasing water in the process, is a ____.

4. ______________________________ are amino acids that are normally made in the body (nonessential) but become essential under certain circumstances, such as during critical illness.

5. The most abundant fibrous protein in the body is ______________________.

6. The fluid located outside of cells is ______________________________.

7. ______________________________ is a water-insoluble fibrous protein that is the primary constituent of hair, nails, and the outer layer of the skin.

8. ______________________________ is an inherited disorder that causes widespread dysfunction of the exocrine glands resulting in chronic lung disease, abnormally high levels of electrolytes (e.g., sodium, potassium, chloride) in sweat, and deficiency of pancreatic enzymes needed for digestion.

9. A condition resulting from long-term inadequate intakes of protein and energy that can lead to wasting of body tissues and increased susceptibility to infection is ____.

10. The main nitrogen-containing waste product in mammals is ______________. Formed in liver cells from ammonia and carbon dioxide, it is carried via the bloodstream to the kidneys, where it is excreted in the urine.

11. ______________________________ involves a change in the three-dimensional structure of a protein resulting in an unfolded polypeptide chain that cannot fulfill the protein's function.

12. The constant breakdown and synthesis of proteins in the body is called ____.

13. ______________________________ are amino acids the body cannot make at all or cannot make in sufficient quantities to meet the body's needs. These must be supplied in the diet.

14. ______________________________ is the fluid between cells in tissues. It is also called ______________________________.

15. Substances released at the end of a stimulated nerve cell that diffuse across a small gap and bind to another nerve cell or muscle cell, stimulating or inhibiting it, are ______________________________ ______________________________.

16. ______________________________ occurs when nitrogen intake is less than the sum of all sources of nitrogen excretion.

17. ______________________________ occurs when nitrogen intake exceeds the sum of all sources of nitrogen excretion.

18. Amino acids the body can make if supplied with adequate nitrogen are ______________________________ ______________________________. These do not need to be supplied in the diet.

19. ______________________________ is the oxygen-carrying protein that gives blood its red color.

◎ Fill-in-the-Blank Summaries

Amino Acids: The Building Blocks of Protein

Proteins are sequences of amino acids. There are ____________________ different amino acids; ______________________________ are essential and ______________________________ are nonessential. ____________________ and cysteine are both considered ______________________________ amino acids. If your intake of methionine is too low, your body needs cysteine from your diet to free methionine for protein formation. People with ______________________________ lack sufficient amounts of an enzyme that converts ______________________________ to tyrosine. These people must carefully monitor the amount of phenylalanine in their diets to avoid problems such as ______________________________ ______________________________.

One amino acid is linked to the next by a ______________________________. When this bond is created, the carboxyl group of one amino acid binds to the amino group of another amino acid. This reaction releases water in the process. An oligopeptide is a chain of ______________________________ __________ amino acids; a polypeptide contains at least ______________________________ amino acids. Acidity, heat, and oxidation can disrupt the chemical forces that stabilize a protein's shape causing it to ______________________________.

Functions of Body Proteins

Proteins have structural and mechanical functions. ______________________________, the most abundant protein in mammals, gives skin and bones their elastic strength. The proteins that turn energy into mechanical work are known as ______________________ proteins. These proteins are also involved in cell division and sperm swimming. Proteins that catalyze chemical reactions without being used up are ______________________. ______________________ are chemical messengers that are made in one part of the body but act on cells in other parts of the body. ______________________ are blood proteins that attack and inactivate bacteria and viruses. If the body does not have enough protein to maintain normal levels of blood proteins, fluids will leak into surrounding tissues and cause edema. Proteins help maintain ______________________ levels in body fluids by serving as buffers; they donate hydrogen ions when conditions are alkaline. They pick up extra hydrogen ions when conditions are acidic and donate hydrogen ions when conditions are alkaline. More than one third of the energy your body uses at rest is consumed by the sodium-potassium protein pump, which controls cell volume and nerve impulses. If the diet does not provide enough energy to sustain vital functions, the body will sacrifice its own protein to make energy and glucose.

Notes

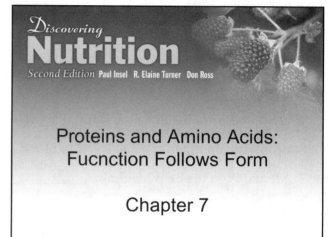

Amino Acids Are the Building Blocks of Protein

- Proteins are sequences of amino acids
- Types of amino acids
  - Essential: must come from diet
  - Nonessential: can be made in the body

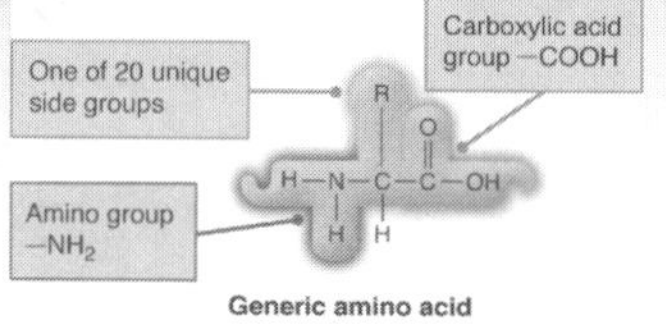

Generic amino acid

Amino Acids Are the Building Blocks of Protein

- Protein structure
  - Chain of amino acids
    - Sequence of amino acids determines shape
    - Shape of protein determines function
  - Denaturing protein structure
    - Disrupts function
    - Caused by heat, acid, oxidation, agitation

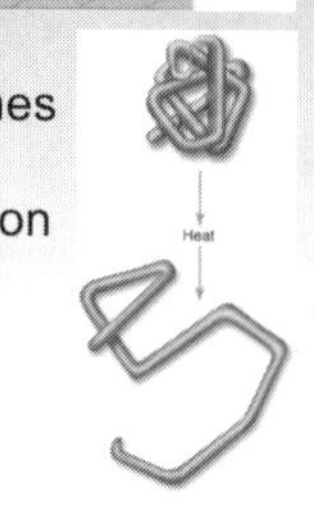

Functions of Body Protein

- Structural and mechanical functions
  - Collagen
  - Keratin
  - Motor proteins
- Enzymes
  - Catalyze reactions
- Hormones
  - Regulate body processes

Structural and Mechanical

Enzymes

Hormones

Functions of Body Protein

- Immune function
  - Antibodies attack bacteria and viruses
- Fluid balance
  - Blood proteins attract fluid
- Acid-base balance
  - Proteins act as buffers
- Transport
  - Lipoproteins, other carrier molecules
- Source of energy
  - 4 kcal/g

Antibodies

Fluid balance

Acid-base balance

Transport

Protein Digestion and Absorption

- Stomach
  - Proteins are denatured by hydrochloric acid
  - Pepsin begins digestion
- Small intestine
  - Pancreatic and intestinal proteases and peptidases complete digestion
  - Amino acids are absorbed into the bloodstream

Notes

Notes

Proteins in the Body

- Protein synthesis
  - Directed by cellular DNA
  - Draws on amino acid pool
- Synthesis of non-protein substances

Proteins in the Body

- Protein and nitrogen excretion
  - Deamination of amino acids
    - Removes nitrogen (amino) group
    - Amino groups converted to urea for excretion

Proteins in the Body

- Nitrogen balance
  - Nitrogen intake vs. nitrogen output
- Nitrogen equilibrium
  - Nitrogen intake = nitrogen output
  - Healthy adults
- Positive nitrogen balance
  - Nitrogen intake > nitrogen output
  - Growth, recovery from illness
- Negative nitrogen balance
  - Nitrogen intake < nitrogen output
  - Injury, illness

Proteins in the Diet

- Recommended protein intake
  - Adult RDA = 0.8 gram per kilogram body weight
  - Infant RDA = ~ 1.5 grams per kilogram body weight
- Increased protein needs
  - Physical stress
  - Injury
  - Intense weight training
- U.S. protein intake > protein needs

Proteins in the Diet

- Protein quality
  - Complete proteins
    - Supply all essential amino acids
    - Animal proteins, soy proteins
  - Incomplete proteins
    - Low in one or more essential amino acids
    - Most plant proteins

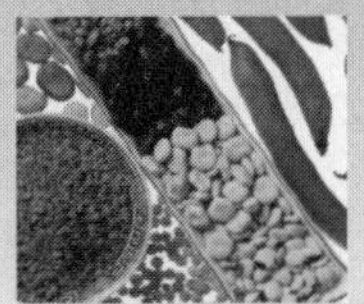

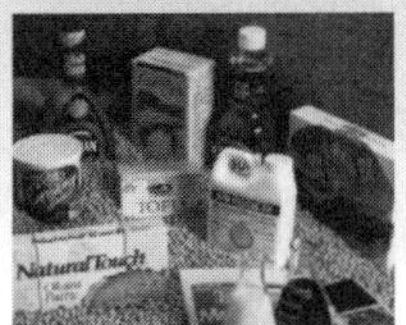

Photos courtesy of the USDA

Proteins in the Diet

- Protein quality
  - Two incomplete proteins = complete protein
  - Complementary proteins

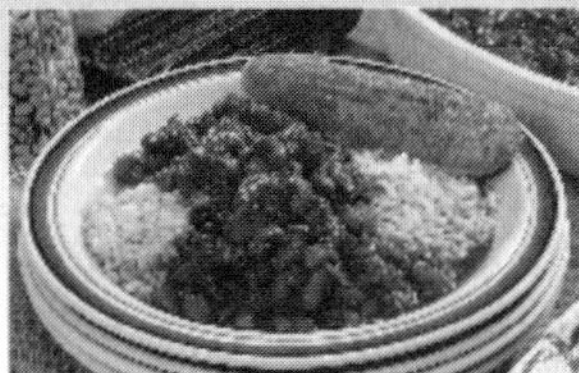

Photo © PhotoDisc

Notes

Notes

Proteins in the Diet

- Evaluating protein quality
  - Amino acid composition
  - Digestibility
  - Protein Digestibility-Corrected Amino Acid Score (PDCAAS)
    - Used to determine %DV

Proteins in the Diet

- Protein and amino acid supplements
  - Generally not needed
  - Risks unknown

The Pros and Cons of Vegetarian Eating

- Types of vegetarian diets
  - Semi-vegetarian
    - Usually includes fish, poultry; no red meat
  - Lacto-ovo vegetarian
    - Includes milk, eggs
  - Vegan
    - Plant foods only

The Pros and Cons of Vegetarian Eating

- Health benefits
  - Less fat, saturated fat, cholesterol intake
    - Reduces risk for heart disease, obesity, hypertension, cancer
- Health risks
  - Vegan diets may be low in some nutrients
    - Calcium, iron, zinc, vitamin D, vitamin B_{12}
  - More restrictive food choices = less nutrients
  - Careful planning needed for growth

The Pros and Cons of Vegetarian Eating

- Dietary recommendations
  - Choose a variety of foods
  - Choose whole, unrefined foods
  - Choose a variety of fruits and vegetables
  - Choose lower-fat dairy products and eggs in moderation
  - Consume a regular source of vitamins B_{12} and D
    - Fortified foods or supplements

The Health Effects of Too Little Protein

- Protein-energy malnutrition (PEM)
  - Kwashiorkor
  - Marasmus

Notes

Notes

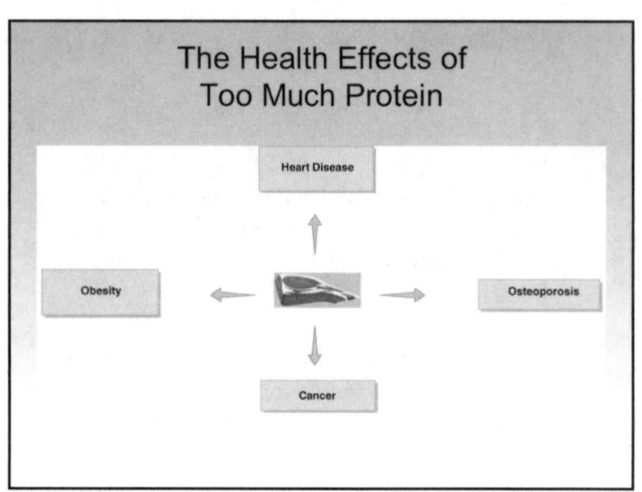
The Health Effects of
Too Much Protein
Heart Disease
Obesity
Osteoporosis
Cancer

SPOTLIGHT ON

Metabolism

The Spotlight outline provides you with an organizational guide to the topics and ideas presented in this section of the text.

Energy: Fuel for Work
- Transferring Food Energy to Cellular Energy

What Is Metabolism?
- The Cell Is the Metabolic Processing Center
- ATP: The Body's Energy Currency
- NAD^+ and FAD: The Body's Transport Shuttles

Breakdown and Release of Energy
- Extracting Energy from Carbohydrate
- Extracting Energy from Fat
- Extracting Energy from Protein

Biosynthesis and Storage
- Making Carbohydrate (Glucose)
- Making Fat (Fatty Acids)
- Making Ketone Bodies
- Making Protein (Amino Acids)

Special States
- Feasting
- Fasting

◎ Key Terms

Define the following terms.

1. **metabolism** ______
2. **acetyl CoA** ______
3. **cells** ______
4. **ketogenesis** ______
5. **aerobic** ______
6. **catabolism** ______
7. **photosynthesis** ______
8. **mitochondria** ______
9. **citric acid cycle** ______
10. **cytosol** ______

11. **organelles** ____

12. **metabolites** ____

13. **chemical energy** ____

14. **biosynthesis** ____

15. **anabolism** ____

16. **cytoplasm** ____

17. **gluconeogenesis** ____

18. **GTP** ____

19. **glycolysis** ____

20. **coenzymes** ____

◎ Fill-in-the-Blank

1. The breakdown of a fatty acid into numerous molecules of the two-carbon compound acetyl coenzyme A (acetyl CoA) is called ____________________.
2. ____________________ is the main direct fuel that cells use to synthesize molecules, contract muscles, transport substances, and perform other tasks.
3. Nicotinamide adenine dinucleotide (NAD^+), a coenzyme derived from the B vitamin niacin, becomes ____________________ as it accepts a pair of high-energy electrons for transport in cells.
4. The three-carbon compound that results from glycolysis is ____________________.
5. ____________________ are compounds required for an enzyme to be active. They include coenzymes and metal ions such as iron, copper, and magnesium.
6. ____________________ is the synthesis of fatty acids from acetyl CoA derived from the metabolism of fats, alcohol, and some amino acids.
7. ____________________ is a four-carbon intermediate compound in the citric acid cycle.
8. The primary site of genetic information in the cell, enclosed in a double-layered membrane, is the ____________________.
9. ____________________ is an organized series of protein carrier molecules located in mitochondrial membranes.
10. ____________________ refers to the absence of oxygen or the ability of a process to occur in the absence of oxygen.

11. ________________ are organic compounds that contain a chemical group consisting of C=O (a carbon–oxygen double bond) bound to two hydrocarbons. Pyruvate and fructose are examples of these.

12. ________________ is a molecule composed of adenosine and two phosphate groups.

13. ________________ is a cofactor derived from the vitamin pantothenic acid.

14. A ________________ is a series of chemical reactions that either break down a large compound into smaller units or synthesize more complex molecules from smaller ones.

15. ________________ is a compound that transports fatty acids from the cytosol into the mitochondria, where they undergo beta-oxidation.

16. A ________________ amino acid breaks down to acetyl CoA.

17. ________________ is a coenzyme derived from the B vitamin riboflavin, which becomes $FADH_2$ as it accepts a pair of high-energy electrons for transport in cells.

18. Acidification of the blood caused by a buildup of ketone bodies is called ________________. It is primarily a consequence of uncontrolled type 1 diabetes mellitus and can be life threatening.

19. The term ________________ describes an amino acid whose carbon skeleton can be used in gluconeogenesis to form glucose.

20. ________________ is a three-carbon compound that is produced when insufficient oxygen is present in cells to break down pyruvate to acetyl CoA.

◎ Fill-in-the-Blank Summaries

Energy: Fuel for Work

Our cells get their energy from ________________ energy held in molecular bonds of carbohydrates, fats, and proteins. Green plants use light energy from the sun to make carbohydrate in a process called ________________. Our bodies extract energy from food in three stages. Stage 1 consists of digestion, absorption, and ________________. Stage 2 includes the breakdown of many small molecules into a few key metabolites. In Stage 3, the complete breakdown of metabolites to water and ________________________ liberates large amounts of energy.

The term ________________________ describes a series of chemical reactions that either break down a large compound (catabolism) or build more complex molecules (anabolism). Cells are known as the "work centers" of metabolism. The basic animal cell is divided into two parts—the ________________________ and the ________________________, which is filled with a fluid called cystosol. The ________________________ are power generators that contain many important energy-producing pathways. ________________________ and their cofactors speed up chemical reactions in metabolic pathways.

Breakdown and Release of Energy

Although each energy-yielding nutrient initially follows a different metabolic pathway, they all follow the ________________________, ________________________, ________________________, and the electron transport chain. During glycolysis one molecule of glucose yields ________________ NADH, a net of two ____________ and ____________ pyruvate. In the next step of carbohydrate metabolism, pyruvate is converted to ________________. Without oxygen, pyruvate cannot be converted to this substance. In this case, it is rerouted to form ________________________. ________________________ begins when acetyl CoA combines with oxaloacetate to yield citrate. This cycle produces most of the energy-rich molecules that ultimately generate ATP. It is also an important source of building blocks for fatty acids and ________________________.

The electron transport chain is the last step in glucose breakdown and occurs in the inner ________________________ membrane. Molecules of ________________ produced in the citric acid cycle deliver their high-energy electrons to the beginning of the chain. At the end of the chain, oxygen accepts the energy depleted electrons and then reacts with hydrogen to form water. The three end products of glucose catabolism are water, ________________________, and ATP.

Special States: Fasting

When your body is faced with starvation it must deal with several dilemmas. The first priority is to preserve glucose-dependent tissue: ________________________, brain cells, and the central nervous system. After carbohydrate reserves are depleted within a few hours, circulating ________________________ are used to make glucose and ________________________. The second priority is to maintain muscle mass. Because little glucose can be made from triglycerides stored in the adipose tissue, the brain cells adapt so that they can use ______________________ for fuel.

When glucose levels drop to baseline levels after several hours of fasting, the hormone ______________ ______________ stimulates the breakdown of liver glycogen to glucose. During the first few days of starvation glucogenic amino acids, especially alanine, furnish 90% of the brain's glucose supply, and ________________________ provide(s) the remaining 10%. Eventually protein breakdown must slow down or the body will not survive for more than three weeks without food. Fat catabolism rates double to supply fatty acids for fuel and glycerol for glucose. The average person has ______________ weeks of fat stores; then the body must turn back to protein for energy. Protein breakdown slows drastically and gluconeogenesis drops by two-thirds or more. A starving person can survive until ________________ _______ % of his or her proteins are broken down.

Notes

Discovering **Nutrition**

Second Edition Paul Insel R. Elaine Turner Don Ross

Spotlight on Metabolism

Energy: Fuel for Work

- Energy source
  - Chemical energy in carbohydrates, fat, protein
- Food energy to cellular energy
  - Stage 1: digestion, absorption, transport
  - Stage 2: breakdown of molecules
  - Stage 3: transfer of energy to a form cells can use

What Is Metabolism?

- Catabolism
  - Reactions that break down compounds into small units

What Is Metabolism?

- Anabolism
  - Reactions that build complex molecules from smaller ones

ANABOLIC REACTIONS

Glucose + Glucose → Glycogen (Energy)

Glycerol + Fatty acids → Triglyceride (Energy)

Amino acid + Amino acid → Protein (Energy)

What Is Metabolism?

- Cell is the metabolic processing center
  - Nucleus
  - Cytoplasm: cytosol + organelles
    - Mitochondria are the source of many energy pathways

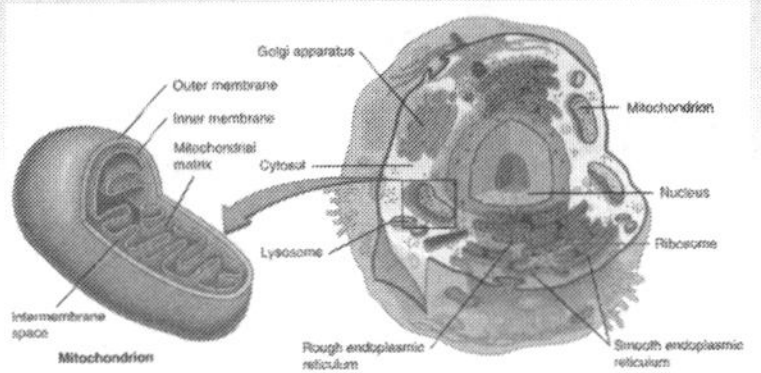

What Is Metabolism?

- ATP is the body's energy currency
  - ATP = adenosine triphosphate
  - Form of energy cells use
- NAD and FAD: transport shuttles
  - Accept high-energy electrons for use in ATP production

ATP, ADP, AND HIGH-ENERGY PHOSPHATE BONDS

ATP: adenosine triphosphate

Adenosine — P_i ~ P_i ~ P_i

Inorganic phosphate group

2 high-energy bonds

Notes

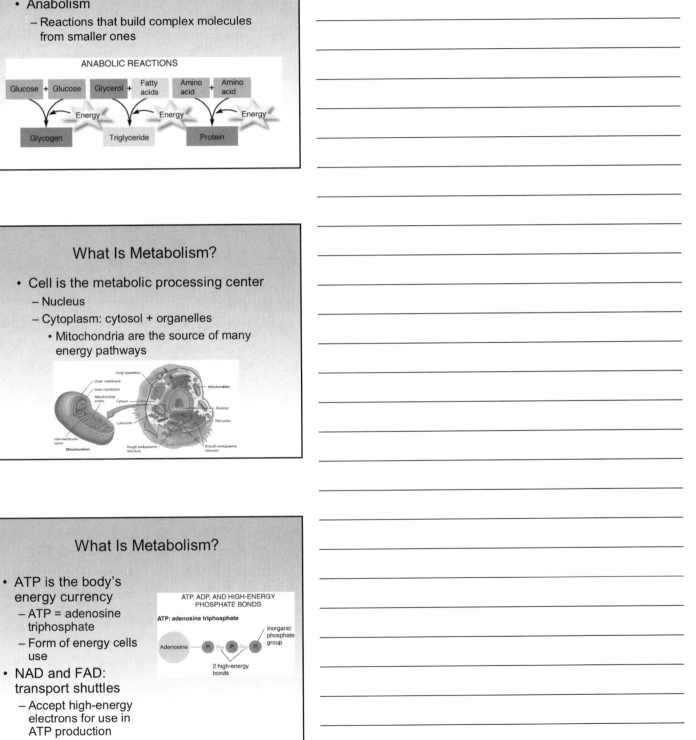

Notes

Extracting Energy

EXTRACTION OF ENERGY

Protein (amino acids) | Carbohydrates (sugars) | Fats (fatty acids)

Energy

Breakdown and Release of Energy

- Extracting energy from carbohydrate
  - Glycolysis
    - Pathway splits glucose into two pyruvates
    - Transfers electrons to NAD
    - Produces some ATP
  - Pyruvate to acetyl CoA
    - Releases CO_2
    - Transfers electrons to NAD

Breakdown and Release of Energy

- Extracting energy from carbohydrate
  - Citric acid cycle
    - Releases CO_2
    - Produces GTP (like ATP)
    - Transfers electrons to NAD and FAD
  - Electron transport chain
    - Accepts electrons from NAD and FAD
    - Produces large amounts of ATP
    - Produces water
  - End products of glucose breakdown
    - ATP, H_2O, CO_2

Breakdown and Release of Energy

- Extracting energy from fat
  - Split triglycerides into glycerol and fatty acids
  - Beta-oxidation
    - Breaks apart fatty acids into acetyl CoA
    - Transfers electrons to NAD and FAD
  - Citric acid cycle
    - Acetyl CoA from beta-oxidation enters cycle
  - Electron transport chain
  - End products of fat breakdown
    - ATP, H_2O, CO_2

Breakdown and Release of Energy

- Extracting energy from protein
  - Split protein into amino acids
  - Split off amino group
    - Converted to urea for excretion
  - Carbon skeleton enters breakdown pathways
  - End products
    - ATP, H_2O, CO_2, urea

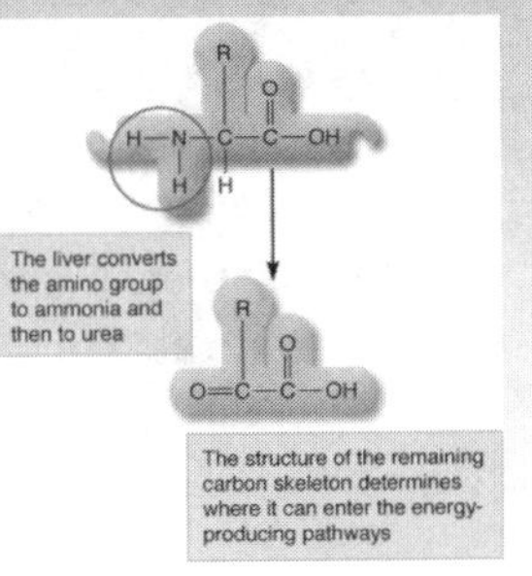

The liver converts the amino group to ammonia and then to urea
The structure of the remaining carbon skeleton determines where it can enter the energy-producing pathways

Breakdown and Release of Energy

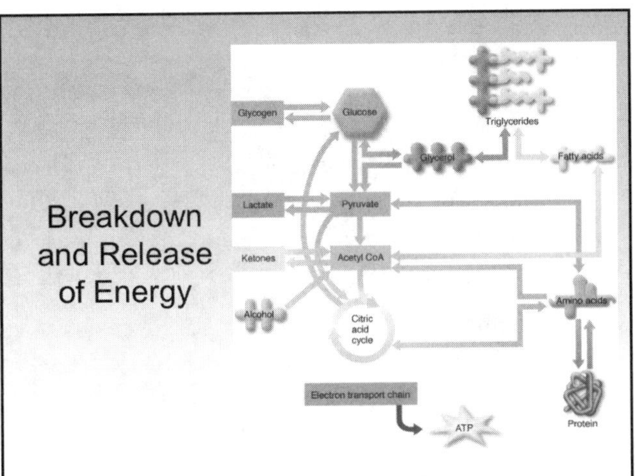

Notes

Notes

Biosynthesis and Storage

- Making carbohydrate (glucose)
  - Gluconeogenesis
    - Uses pyruvate, lactate, glycerol, certain amino acids
- Storing carbohydrate (glycogen)
  - Liver, muscle make glycogen from glucose
- Making fat (fatty acids)
  - Lipogenesis
    - Uses acetyl CoA from fat, amino acids, glucose
- Storing fat (triglyceride)
  - Stored in adipose tissue

Biosynthesis and Storage

- Making ketone bodies (ketogenesis)
  - Made from acetyl CoA
    - When inadequate glucose in cells
- Making protein (amino acids)
  - Amino acid pool supplied from
    - Diet, protein breakdown, cell synthesis

Special States

- Feasting
  - Excess energy intake from carbohydrate, fat, protein
    - Promotes storage

Special States

- Fasting
  - Inadequate energy intake
    - Promotes breakdown
  - Prolonged fasting
    - Protects body protein as long as possible

! FUEL PRIORITY ! GLUCOSE FOR THE BRAIN

Fuel use shifts to fatty acids and ketone bodies

Protein breakdown supplies glucose for brain function

Fat breakdown is early & rapid to preserve structural proteins

As fat stores are used up, protein breakdown accelerates

Protein

Fat

Carbohydrate

Quantities of stored fuel (kilograms)

Weeks of starvation

Notes

CHAPTER 8

Energy Balance and Weight Management: Finding Your Equilibrium

The chapter outline provides you with an organizational guide to the topics and ideas presented in this chapter of the text.

Energy In
- Hunger, Satiation, and Satiety
- Appetite
- Control by Committee

Energy Out: Fuel Uses
- Major Components of Energy Expenditure
- Estimating Total Energy Expenditure
- DRIs for Energy: Estimated Energy Requirements

Body Composition: Understanding Fatness and Weight

Assessing Body Weight

Assessing Body Fatness

Body Fat Distribution

Overweight and Obesity
- Factors in the Development of Obesity
- Health Risks of Overweight and Obesity

Weight Management
- The Perception of Weight
- What Goals Should I Set?
- Adopting a Healthy Weight-Management Lifestyle
- Diet and Eating Habits
- Thinking and Emotions
- Weight-Management Approaches

Underweight
- Causes and Assessment
- Weight-Gain Strategies

Key Terms

Define the following terms.

1. appetite ______________________________
2. extreme obesity ______________________________
3. waist circumference ______________________________
4. energy balance ______________________________
5. leptin ______________________________
6. sleep apnea ______________________________
7. hypothalamus ______________________________

8. **basal energy expenditure (BEE)** ______________________________

9. **gynoid obesity** ______________________________

10. **hunger** ______________________________

11. **body mass index (BMI)** ______________________________

12. **built environment** ______________________________

13. **energy intake** ______________________________

14. **basal metabolic rate (BMR)** ______________________________

15. **energy equilibrium** ______________________________

16. **android obesity** ______________________________

17. **energy output** ______________________________

18. **negative self-talk** ______________________________

19. **resting energy expenditure (REE)** ______________________________

20. **body fat distribution** ______________________________

21. **lean body mass** ______________________________

22. **total energy expenditure (TEE)** ______________________________

23. **satiation** ______________________________

24. **metabolic fitness** ______________________________

25. **skinfold measurements** ______________________________

26. **satiety** ______________________________

◎ Fill-in-the-Blank

1. The ______________________________ is a behavioral model that includes the external and internal events that precede and follow the behavior. This involves antecedents and the events that precede the behavior, followed by consequences that positively or negatively reinforce the behavior.

2. Constructive mental or verbal statements made to one's self to change a belief or behavior are called ______________________________.

3. A ______________________________ is a device used to measure the density of the body based on the volume of air displaced as a person sits in a sealed chamber of known volume.

4. A person is ______________________________ if they have a BMI less than 18.5 kg/m^2.

5. Obesity due to an above-average number of fat cells is called ______________________________ ______________________________.

6. ______________________________ are individuals who routinely consume a very large amount of food in a brief period of time (e.g., two hours) and lose control over how much and what is eaten.

7. Individuals who routinely avoid food as long as possible and then gorge on food are ______________________________ ______________________________.

8. The output of energy associated with fidgeting, maintenance of posture, and other minimal physical exertions is ______________________________.

9. A person is ______________________________ if their BMI is at or above 25 kg/m^2 and less than 30 kg/m^2.

10. Obesity due to an increase in both the size and number of fat cells is called ______________________________ ______________________________.

11. ______________________________ is a neurotransmitter widely distributed throughout the brain and peripheral nervous tissue. Its activity has been linked to eating behavior, depression, anxiety, and cardiovascular function.

12. Repeated periods of gaining and losing weight is called ______________________________.

13. ______________________________ occurs when energy intake is lower than energy expenditure, resulting in a depletion of body energy stores and weight loss.

14. ______________________________ is a clinical measure of resting energy expenditure performed three to four hours after eating or performing significant physical activity.

15. ______________________________ is a technique used to estimate amounts of total body water, lean tissue mass, and total body fat. It uses the resistance of tissue to the flow of an alternating electric current.

16. ______________________________ occurs when a person has a BMI at or above 30 kg/m^2.

17. Obesity due to an increase in the size of fat cells is ______________________________ ______________________________.

18. ______________________________ is a hormone produced by the stomach that stimulates feeding by increasing release of neuropeptide Y.

19. ______________________________ is defined as having a BMI at or above 18.5 kg/m^2 and less than 25 kg/m^2.

20. Diets supplying 400 to 800 kilocalories per day, which include adequate high-quality protein, little or no fat, and little carbohydrate are called ______________________________ ______________________________.

21. Determining body density by measuring the volume of water displaced when the body is fully submerged in a specialized water tank is called ______________________________ ______________________________.

22. The ______________________________ is the energy used to digest, absorb, and metabolize energy-yielding foodstuffs. It constitutes about 10 percent of total energy expenditure but is influenced by various factors.

23. The adoption of healthful and sustainable eating and exercise behaviors that reduce disease risk and improve well-being is ______________________________.

24. ______________________________ occurs when energy intake exceeds energy expenditure, resulting in an increase in body energy stores and weight gain.

25. ______________________________ is the chemical or anatomical composition of the body. It is commonly defined as the proportions of fat, muscle, bone, and other tissues in the body.

◎ Fill-in-the-Blank Summaries

Energy In

There are three processes that influence eating. ______________________________ is the first process followed by ______________________________, which lets you know that you are full. The final process, ______________________________, determines the interval between meals. The difference between hunger and appetite is that hunger is a(n) ______________________________ for food while appetite is the ______________________________ for food.

______________________________ tend to delay satiation and encourage overeating. ______________________________ tend to enhance satiety by slowing gastric emptying and enhance satiation with their bulking properties. Overall energy availability is a more important regulator than circulating nutrient levels.

Exposure to ______________________________ tends to increase the amount we eat; exposure to ______________________________ tends to reduce it. NPY is a neuroendocrine factor that triggers decreased energy expenditure and increased food intake. It stimulates a desire to eat rather than a desire for energy. Fat cells produce ____________________________________, which tells the central nervous system how much fat the body is storing.

Energy Out

The minimum energy necessary to sustain life is called the ______________________________________. This type of energy is measured as either the basal metabolic rate or the ______________________________________. Over time, a person's RMR varies by less than 5%. A person's RMR ______________________ as they age, because some lean tissue is replaced by fat. Lean tissue has ____ metabolic activity than fat tissue.

Energy costs of physical activity depend on the activity's type, ______________________________, and intensity. The energy associated with fidgeting and maintenance of posture is called ______________________________.

The energy output our bodies expend while digesting, absorbing, and metabolizing nutrients is collectively called the thermic effect of food. The TEF is lowest for ____ and highest for ____________________________________. Typically, TEF accounts for approximately _____________________________ of total energy expenditure.

Body Composition

The National Institutes of Health released guidelines in 1998 that define obesity in adults as a BMI of greater than ________________________________ kg/m^2. The BMI has a limited ability to distinguish between muscle weight and excess fat weight. Densitometry is the measure of body density. In ________________________________, body density is calculated using the above-water weight, the submerged weight and, the quantity of water displaced during submersion. Done correctly, body composition estimates from skinfold thickness measurements correlate well with ____. This type of measurement is especially useful in tracking changes to subcutaneous fat distribution over time. Body fat distribution can be a risk factor for heart disease and diabetes. ______________________________________ obesity is more common in ____ and refers to excess fat being distributed around the hips and thighs. ________________ obesity is more common in _____________________________________ and has excess fat distributed around the abdomen.

Notes

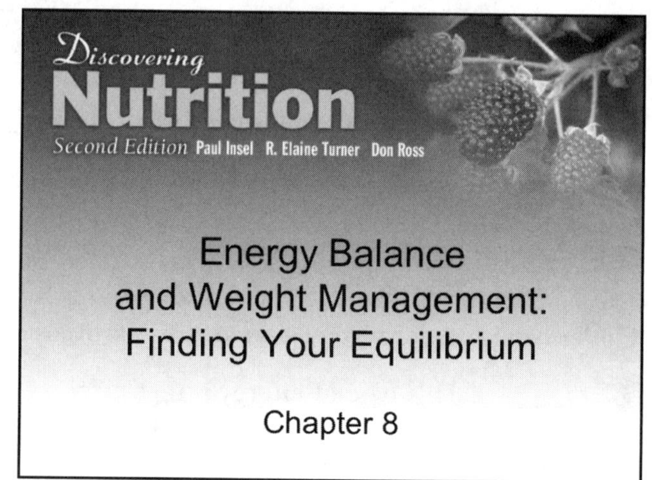

Discovering
Nutrition
Second Edition Paul Insel R. Elaine Turner Don Ross
Energy Balance
and Weight Management:
Finding Your Equilibrium
Chapter 8

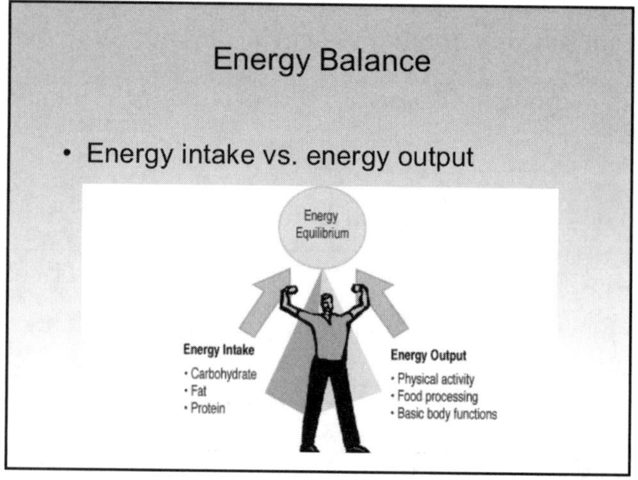

Energy Balance

- Energy equilibrium
  - Intake = output
  - Maintain weight
- Positive energy balance
  - Intake > output
  - Gain weight
- Negative energy balance
  - Intake < output
  - Lose weight

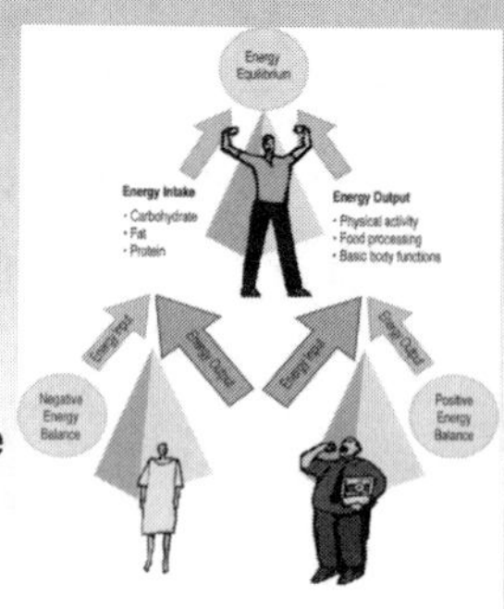

Energy In

- Regulation of intake
  - Hunger
    - Prompts eating; physiological desire
  - Satiation
    - Signals to stop eating
  - Satiety
    - Lack of hunger
  - Appetite
    - Psychological desire

Hunger signals you to begin eating
Growing hunger
I'm beginning to get hungry
Let's eat
Between meals
Eating
I'm full
Satiety is the satisfaction between meals
Satiation signals you to stop eating

Energy In: Regulatory Factors

Internal and external factors
Stress
Mood
Internal factors that influence hunger
Digestive organ functions
Central nervous system functions
Conditions such as anorexia nervosa, trauma, infection
Temperature
Drug effects
Metabolic influences (hormones and neurotransmitters)
External factors that influence appetite
Social situation
Time of day
Sensory properties of food
Cultural background
Environment: social and climatic

Energy Out: Fuel Uses

- Major components of energy expenditure
  - Resting energy expenditure (REE)
    - Energy for basic body functions
    - Affected by body size, composition, age, gender

Thermic effect of food (~10%)
Physical activity (15–30%)
Resting energy expenditure (60–75%)

Notes

Notes

Energy Out: Fuel Uses

- Major components of energy expenditure
  - Physical activity
    - Highly variable
    - Affected by body size fitness level, type of activity
  - Thermic effect of food (TEF)
    - Energy to digest, absorb, metabolize food

Estimating Energy Expenditure

- Resting energy expenditure (REE)
  - 1.0 kcal/kg/hr for males
  - 0.9 kcal/kg/hr for females
- Physical activity
  - Add a % of REE (see Table 8.2)
- Thermic effect of food
  - 5% to 10% of (REE + physical activity)

Estimating Energy Expenditure

- Estimated Energy Requirement (EER)
  - Equations for males and females
    - Factors for age, weight, height, physical activity
  - Predicts total energy expenditure (TEE)

Notes

Body Composition: Understanding Fatness and Weight

- Assessing body weight
  - Body mass index (BMI)
    - Weight (kg) $\prod$ height^2 (m)
    - BMI < 18.5 kg/m^2 = underweight
    - BMI 18.5 to < 25 kg/m^2 = normal weight
    - BMI 25 to < 30kg/m^2 = overweight
    - BMI ≥ 30 kg/m^2 = obese

Body Composition: Understanding Fatness and Weight

- Assessing body fatness
  - Underwater weighing
  - Bioelectrical impedance
  - Skinfold measurements

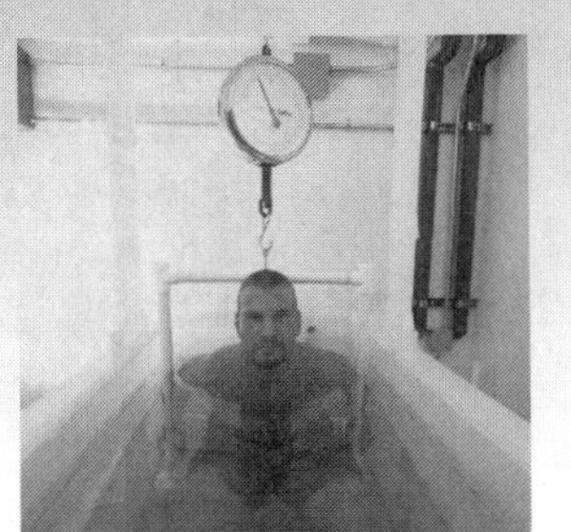

Body Composition: Understanding Fatness and Weight

- Body fat distribution
  - Waist circumference
  - Gynoid obesity (“pear”)
    - Excess fat in hips and thighs
  - Android obesity (“apple”)
    - Excess fat around abdomen

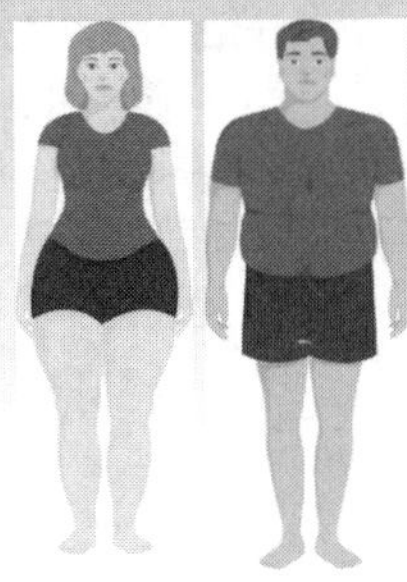

Notes

Overweight and Obesity

- Major public health problem
- Factors in development of obesity
  - Biological
    - Heredity and genetics
    - Fat cell development
    - Sex and age
    - Race and ethnicity

Overweight and Obesity

- Factors in development of obesity
  - Environmental
    - Socioeconomic status
    - Built environment
    - Social factors
  - Lifestyle and behavioral
    - Physical activity
    - Psychological factors

Overweight and Obesity

- Health risks of overweight and obesity
  - Heart disease and stroke
  - Hypertension
  - Diabetes
  - Cancer
  - Joint diseases

Weight Management

- Perception of weight
- Setting realistic goals
- Weight-management lifestyle
  - Diet and eating habits
    - Reduce total calories
    - Reduce fat calories
    - Increase complex carbohydrates
    - Improve eating habits
  - Increase physical activity
  - Stress management
  - Self-acceptance

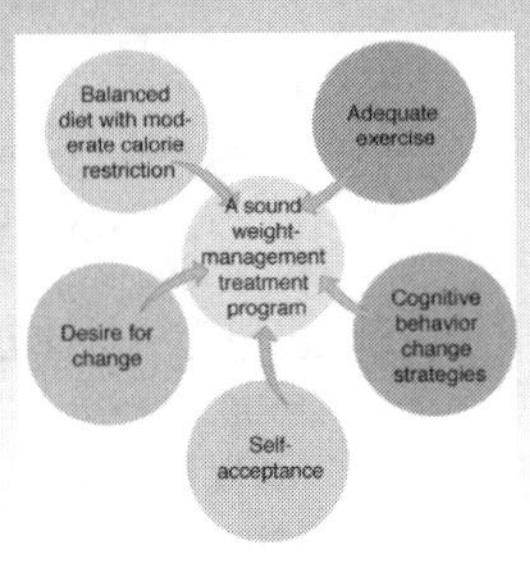

Weight Management

- Weight-management approaches
  - Self-help books and manuals
    - Watch for signs of a fad diet
  - Meal replacements
  - Self-help groups
  - Commercial programs
  - Professional counselors

Weight Management

- Weight-management approaches
  - Prescription drugs
  - OTC drugs and dietary supplements
  - Surgery

Vertical-banded gastroplasty
Surgery reduces stomach capacity by creating a small pouch

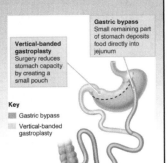

Gastric bypass
Small remaining part of stomach deposits food directly into jejunum

Key
Gastric bypass
Vertical-banded gastroplasty

Notes

Notes

Underweight

- Causes and assessment
  - Illness
  - Eating disorders
  - Metabolic factors
- Weight-gain strategies
  - Small, frequent meals
  - Fluids between meals
  - High-calorie foods and beverages

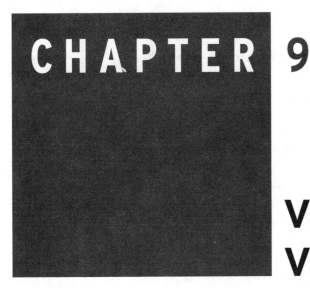

CHAPTER 9

Vitamins: Vital Keys to Health

The chapter outline provides you with an organizational guide to the topics and ideas presented in this chapter of the text.

Understanding Vitamins
- Fat-Soluble Versus Water-Soluble Vitamins
- Vitamins in Foods

Fat-Soluble Vitamins A, D, E, K, and the Carotenoids

Vitamin A: The Retinoids
- Forms of Vitamin A
- Functions of Vitamin A
- Dietary Recommendations for Vitamin A
- Sources of Vitamin A
- Vitamin A Deficiency
- Vitamin A Toxicity

The Carotenoids
- Functions of Carotenoids
- Food Sources, Absorption, and Storage of Carotenoids
- Carotenoid Supplementation

Vitamin D
- Forms and Formation of Vitamin D
- Functions of Vitamin D
- Dietary Recommendations for Vitamin D
- Sources of Vitamin D
- Vitamin D Deficiency
- Vitamin D Toxicity

Vitamin E
- Forms of Vitamin E
- Functions of Vitamin E
- Dietary Recommendations for Vitamin E
- Sources of Vitamin E
- Vitamin E Deficiency
- Vitamin E Toxicity

Vitamin K
- Functions of Vitamin K
- Dietary Recommendations for Vitamin K
- Sources of Vitamin K
- Vitamin K Deficiency
- Vitamin K Toxicity

The Water-Soluble Vitamins: Eight Bs and a C

Thiamin
- Functions of Thiamin
- Dietary Recommendations and Sources of Thiamin
- Thiamin Deficiency
- Thiamin Toxicity

Riboflavin
- Functions of Riboflavin
- Dietary Recommendations and Sources of Riboflavin
- Riboflavin Deficiency
- Riboflavin Toxicity

Niacin
- Functions of Niacin
- Dietary Recommendations and Sources of Niacin
- Niacin Deficiency
- Niacin Toxicity and Medicinal Uses of Niacin

Vitamin B_6
- Functions of Vitamin B_6
- Dietary Recommendations and Sources of Vitamin B_6
- Vitamin B_6 Deficiency
- Vitamin B_6 Toxicity and Medicinal Uses of Vitamin B_6

Folate
- Functions of Folate
- Dietary Recommendations and Sources of Folate
- Folate Deficiency
- Folate Toxicity

Vitamin B_{12}
- Functions of Vitamin B_{12}
- Dietary Recommendations and Sources of Vitamin B_{12}
- Absorption of Vitamin B_{12}
- Vitamin B_{12} Deficiency
- Vitamin B_{12} Toxicity

Pantothenic Acid
- Functions of Pantothenic Acid
- Dietary Recommendations and Sources of Pantothenic Acid
- Pantothenic Acid Deficiency
- Pantothenic Acid Toxicity

Biotin
- Functions of Biotin
- Dietary Recommendations and Sources of Biotin
- Biotin Deficiency
- Biotin Toxicity

Vitamin C
- Functions of Vitamin C
- Dietary Recommendations and Sources of Vitamin C
- Vitamin C Deficiency
- Vitamin C Toxicity

Choline: A Vitamin-Like Substance

Conditional Nutrients and Bogus Vitamins
- Bogus Vitamins

Key Terms

Define the following terms.

1. **cornea** ____________________
2. **glossitis** ____________________
3. **osteoporosis** ____________________
4. **xerophthalmia** ____________________
5. **provitamins** ____________________
6. **spina bifida** ____________________
7. **beriberi** ____________________
8. **keratin** ____________________
9. **rickets** ____________________
10. **myelin sheath** ____________________
11. **anemia** ____________________
12. **osteomalacia** ____________________
13. **retinoids** ____________________
14. **bleaching process** ____________________

15. **cone cells** ______

16. **cheilosis** ______

17. **iodopsin** ______

18. **epithelial tissues** ______

19. **avidin** ______

20. **dark adaptation** ______

21. **carotenoids** ______

22. **menaquinones** ______

23. **retina** ______

24. **teratogen** ______

25. **niacin equivalents (NE)** ______

26. **connective tissues** ______

27. **neural tube defects (NTD)** ______

28. **retinal** ______

29. **provitamin A** ______

30. **retinol activity equivalent (RAE)** ______

◎ Fill-in-the-Blank

1. The millions of cells that line and protect the external and internal surfaces of the body are ______ ______. These form epithelial tissues such as skin and mucous membranes.
2. Riboflavin deficiency is called ______.
3. ______ is a selenium-containing enzyme that reduces toxic hydrogen peroxide formed within cells; it works with vitamin E to reduce free radical damage.
4. The form of vitamin K that comes from plant sources is ______ ______; it is also known as vitamin K_1.
5. A symptom of riboflavin deficiency, ______ involves inflammation and cracking at the corners of the mouth.
6. ______ is an amino acid that serves as a niacin precursor in the body.

7. The active form of vitamin D, ________________________________, is an important regulator of blood calcium levels.

8. ________________________________ is a type of neural tube birth defect in which part or all of the brain is missing.

9. ________________________________ is a medicinal form of vitamin K; it is also known as vitamin K_3.

10. A protein that combines with retinal to form rhodopsin in rod cells is ________________.

11. The inability of the eyes to adjust to dim light or to regain vision quickly after exposure to a flash of bright light is called ________________.

12. ________________________________ is the chemical name for vitamin E. There are four kinds (alpha, beta, gamma, delta), but only alpha is active in the body.

13. Found in rod cells, ________________________________ is a light-sensitive pigment molecule that consists of a protein called opsin combined with retinal.

14. Formative cells whose daughter cells may differentiate into other cell types are ________________ ________________.

15. Light-sensitive cells in the retina that react to dim light and transmit black-and-white images are ________________________________.

16. ________________________________ is a hormone secreted by the thyroid gland in response to elevated blood calcium. It stimulates calcium deposition in bone and calcium excretion by the kidneys, thus reducing blood calcium.

17. ________________________________ is a form of anemia that results from an autoimmune disorder that damaged cells lining the stomach and inhibited vitamin B_{12} absorption; it causes vitamin B_{12} deficiency.

18. ________________________________ is a type of neural tube birth defect in which the brain is abnormally small.

19. ________________________________ are a measure of folate intake used to account for the high bioavailability of folic acid taken as a supplement compared with the lower bioavailability of the folate found in foods.

20. An outdated system to measure vitamin activity, ________________________________ ________________ does not consider differences in bioavailability.

21. ________________________________ is characterized by excess amounts of megaloblasts in the blood caused by deficiency of folate or vitamin B_{12}.

22. The alcohol form of vitamin A is ______________________________.

23. ______________________________ is a coenzyme of which the vitamin thiamin is a part. It plays a key role in removing carboxyl groups and helps drive the reaction that forms acetyl CoA from pyruvate during metabolism.

24. Anemia characterized by small, pale red blood cells that lack adequate hemoglobin to carry oxygen is ______________________________.

25. The ______________________________ is a hormone secreted by the parathyroid glands in response to low blood calcium. It stimulates calcium release from bone and calcium absorption by the intestines, while decreasing calcium excretion by the kidneys.

26. ______________________________ and tocopherols are collectively known as vitamin E.

27. The acid form of vitamin A is ______________________________.

28. A symptom of riboflavin deficiency, ______________________________ is a disease of the oil-producing glands of the skin.

◎ Fill-in-the-Blank Summaries

Vitamin A

The body uses ______________________________ active forms of vitamin A, known collectively as the ______________________________. While all forms have essential functions, ______________________________ is the key player in the vitamin A family. In well-nourished people, the ______________________________ stores more than 90% of the body's vitamin A. The remainder is stored in adipose tissue, lungs, and kidneys. Vitamin A is important to vision. In the eye, retinal combines with opsin to form a pigment called ______________________________, which makes it possible to see in dim light. Vitamin A is also involved in color vision as part of the pigment in ______________________________. A lack of vitamin A affects rod cells first so as a vitamin A deficiency worsens ______________________________ emerges before ______________________________. A large proportion of the body's vitamin A is in the form of retinoic acid. It is involved in cell differentiation, the process when ______________________________ develop into specific types of cells with unique functions. The best sources of provitamin A carotenoids are dark green and ______________________________ vegetables. Vitamin A deficiency is the leading cause of ______________________________ in the world.

Vitamin D

The body can synthesize all of the vitamin D it needs with just sufficient amounts of ____________________ ___________. Vitamin D is considered both a vitamin and a ____________________________. Adequate vitamin D prevents a childhood disease called ______________________________. The liver and adipose tissue store vitamin D. When it is needed the liver and kidneys convert stored vitamin D to ______________________________, which works with parathyroid hormone and _____________ __________________________ from the thyroid gland to regulate blood calcium levels. Other than fortified products, good amounts of vitamin D can also be found in ______________________________ _______. In the United States, rickets is sometimes seen in children who have ___________________. ______________________________ is a related skeletal problem seen in adults with a vitamin D deficiency that results in softened bones and bending of the spine.

Vitamin C

Vitamin C plays an important role in the formation of the most abundant protein in the human body ______________________________. Like vitamin E, Vitamin C works as an __________________ _____________. Vitamin C is needed to synthesize many essential substances. The first signs of scurvy arise after ______________________________ of a vitamin C free diet. Scurvy is _________ ______________________________ in developed countries. Less severe signs of inadequate vitamin C intake are ______________________________ and ______________________________. If a healthy person consumes more than _______________ mg of vitamin C a day for a prolonged period of time this may lead to nausea, abdominal cramps, and nosebleeds. Vitamin C has been reputed to prevent or cure ______________________________.

Notes

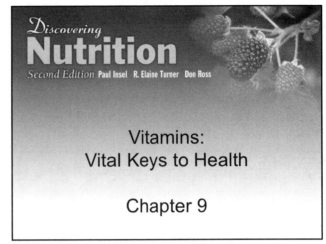

Understanding Vitamins

- Vitamins
  - Organic compounds
  - Needed in small amounts from the diet
  - Regulate body processes

MAJOR ROLES OF VITAMINS

Antioxidants
Vitamin E
Vitamin C

Coenzymes
The 8 B-vitamins

Bone health
Vitamin D
Vitamin K

Vision
Vitamin A

Blood clotting
Vitamin K

Understanding Vitamins

- Fat-soluble vs. water-soluble
  - Fat-soluble: vitamins A, D, E, K
    - Absorbed like fat, into lymphatic system
    - Stored in larger quantities
    - Less vulnerable to cooking losses
  - Water-soluble: 8 B vitamins, vitamin C
    - Absorbed into bloodstream
    - Stored in small amounts
    - Vulnerable to cooking losses

Notes

Understanding Vitamins

- Vitamins in foods
  - Natural sources: all food groups
  - Enriched and fortified foods

Vitamin A

- Functions
  - Vision, cell development and health, immunity
- Food sources
  - Preformed vitamin A: liver, milk, egg yolks
  - Beta-carotene: yellow/orange fruits and vegetables

A
Vision
Cell differentiation
Immunity
Reproduction
Growth

Vitamin A

Excess
Death
Liver damage
Bone fracture
Skin disorders
Birth defects

Vitamin A

A
Adequate intake

Deficiency
Night blindness
Xerophthalmia
Hyperkeratosis
Infection
Death

- Deficiency
  - Affects eyes, skin and other epithelial tissues
- Toxicity
  - Can be fatal

Vitamin D

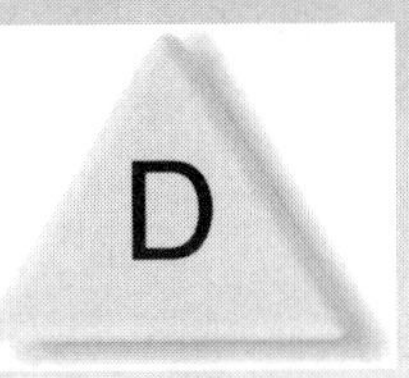

- Synthesis
  - Made in the skin from cholesterol
  - Activated in liver and kidney
- Functions
  - Regulates blood calcium levels
- Food sources
  - Fortified milk, fortified cereals

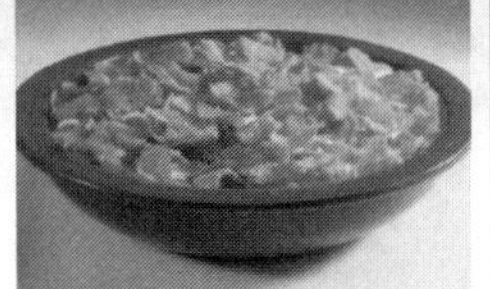

Vitamin D

- Deficiency
  - Rickets in children
  - Osteomalacia and osteoporosis in adults
- Toxicity
  - Hypercalcemia

North of 42 degrees latitude, sunlight is too weak to synthesize vitamin D from late October through early March. The same effect occurs during the winter in the southern hemisphere south of 42 degrees latitude

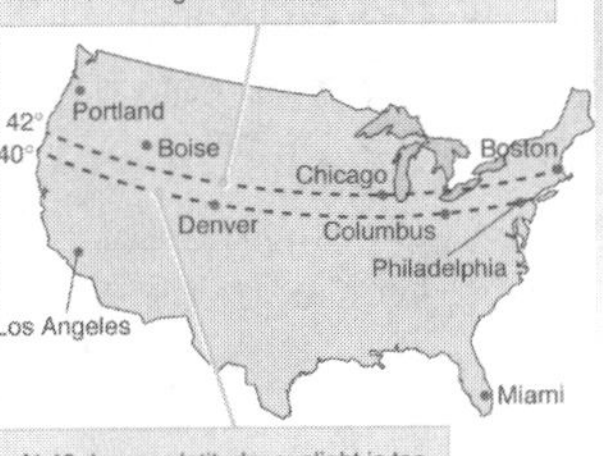

At 40 degrees latitude, sunlight is too weak to synthesize vitamin D during January and February

Vitamin E

- Functions
  - Antioxidant
    - Protects cell membranes from free radicals

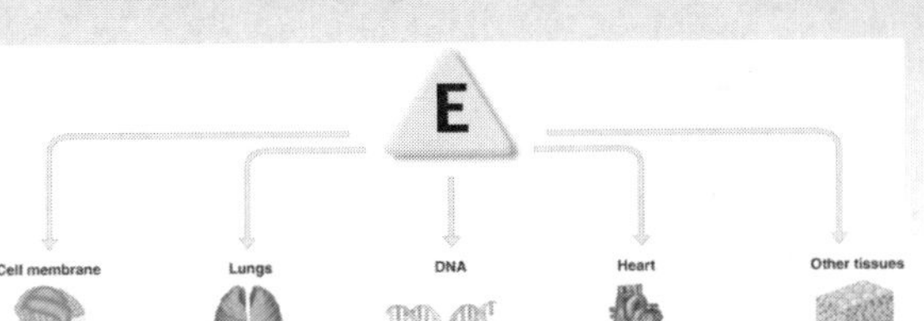

Notes

Notes

Vitamin E

- Food sources
  - Nuts and seeds
  - Wheat germ
  - Oils, margarine, salad dressing
- Deficiency
  - Hemolysis
- Toxicity is rare

Vitamin K

- Functions
  - Blood clotting
  - Formation of bone
- Food sources
  - Green vegetables, liver, egg yolks

K

Vitamin K

- Deficiency
  - Rare in healthy people
  - Increases risk of hemorrhage
- Excess
  - Can interfere with anticoagulant medications
  - Toxicity is rare

Thiamin

- Functions
  - Coenzyme in energy metabolism
  - Helps synthesize neurotransmitters
- Food sources
  - Whole and enriched grains
  - Pork, legumes, nuts, liver
- Deficiency
  - Beriberi

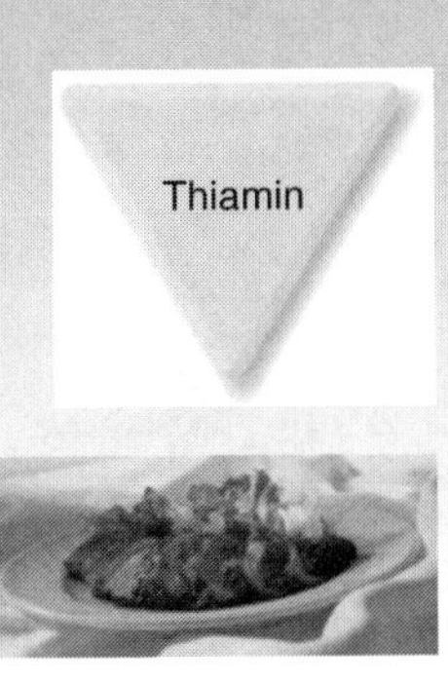

Riboflavin

- Functions
  - Coenzyme in energy metabolism
  - Supports antioxidants
- Food sources
  - Milk and dairy products
  - Whole and enriched grains
- Deficiency
  - Ariboflavinosis

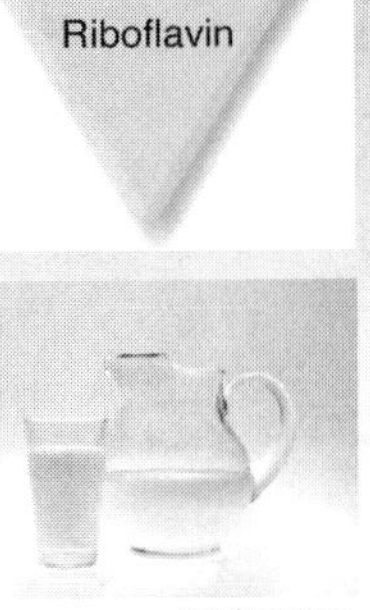

Photo@LiquidLibrary

Niacin

- Functions
  - Coenzyme in energy metabolism
  - Supports fatty acid synthesis
- Food sources
  - Whole and enriched grains
  - Meat, poultry, fish, nuts, and peanuts

Niacin

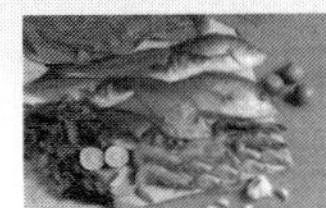

Notes

Notes

Niacin

- Deficiency
  - Pellagra
- Toxicity
  - High doses used to treat high blood cholesterol
  - Side effects: skin flushing, liver damage

Vitamin B_6

- Functions
  - Coenzyme in protein and amino acid metabolism
  - Supports immune system
- Food sources
  - Meat, fish, poultry, liver
  - Potatoes, bananas, sunflower seeds

B6

Photo@DigitalStock

Vitamin B_6

- Deficiency
  - Microcytic hypochromic anemia
- Toxicity
  - Can cause permanent nerve damage in high doses

Folate

- Functions
  - Coenzyme in DNA synthesis and cell division
  - Needed for normal red blood cell synthesis
- Food sources
  - Green leafy vegetables, orange juice, legumes
  - Fortified cereals, enriched grains

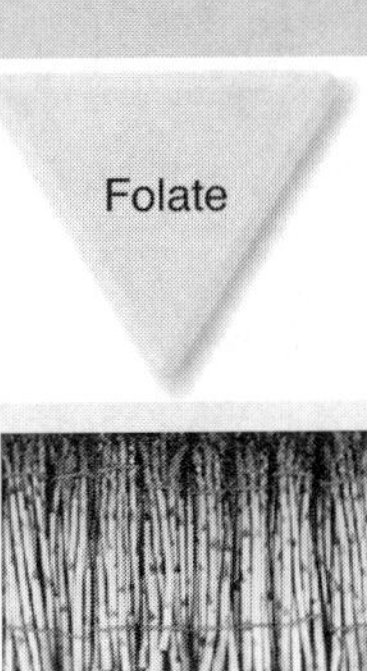

Folate

- Deficiency
  - Megaloblastic anemia
  - Can contribute to neural tube defects
  - Women of childbearing age need 400 micrograms per day of folic acid
- Toxicity
  - Can mask vitamin B_{12} deficiency

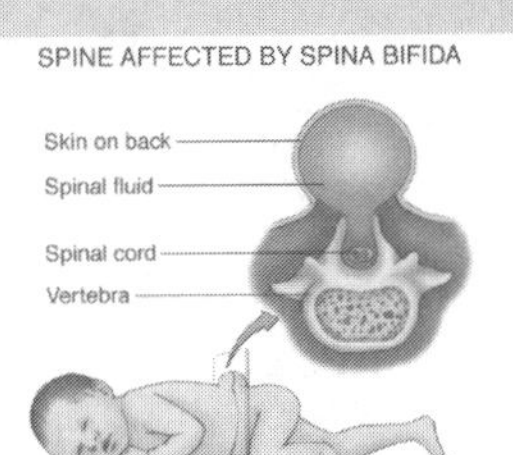

Vitamin B_{12}

- Functions
  - Needed for normal folate function
    - DNA and red blood cell synthesis
  - Maintains myelin sheath around nerves
- Food sources
  - Only animal foods: meats, liver, milk, eggs
- Deficiency
  - Megaloblastic anemia + nerve damage

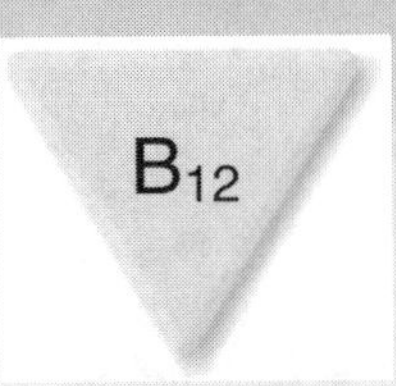

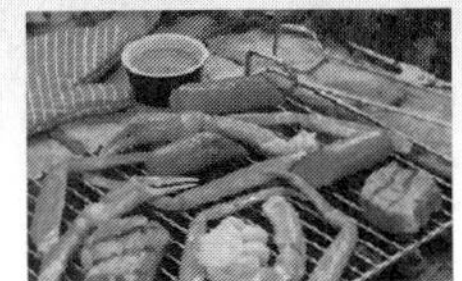

Notes

Notes

Pantothenic Acid

Pantothenic acid

- Functions
  - Component of coenzyme A
- Food sources
  - Widespread in foods
- Deficiency and toxicity are rare

Biotin

Biotin

- Functions
  - Amino acid metabolism
  - Fatty acid synthesis
  - DNA synthesis
- Food sources
  - Cauliflower, liver, peanuts, cheese
- Deficiency and toxicity are rare

Vitamin C

C

- Functions
  - Antioxidant
  - Needed for collagen synthesis
- Food sources
  - Fruits: citrus, strawberries, kiwi
  - Vegetables: broccoli, tomatoes, potatoes

Vitamin C

- Deficiency
  - Scurvy
- Toxicity
  - May cause GI distress in high doses

Notes

SPOTLIGHT ON

Alcohol

The Spotlight outline provides you with an organizational guide to the topics and ideas presented in this section of the text.

History of Alcohol Use
The Character of Alcohol
Alcohol: Is It a Nutrient?
Alcohol and Its Sources
Alcohol Absorption
Alcohol Metabolism
- Metabolizing Small Amounts of Alcohol
- Metabolizing Large Amounts of Alcohol
- Removing Alcohol from Circulation
- Individual Differences in Alcohol Metabolism

When Alcohol Becomes a Problem
- Alcohol in the Brain and the Nervous System
- Alcohol's Effect on the Gastrointestinal System
- Alcohol and the Liver
- Fetal Alcohol Syndrome

Alcoholics and Malnutrition
- Poor Diet
- Vitamin Deficiencies
- Mineral Deficiencies
- Macronutrients
- Body Weight

Does Alcohol Have Benefits?

◎ Key Terms

Define the following terms.

1. **alcohol** ____________________
2. **binge drinking** ____________________
3. **standard drink** ____________________
4. **fatty liver** ____________________
5. **hangover** ____________________
6. **ethanol** ____________________
7. **fetal alcohol syndrome (FAS)** ____________________
8. **French paradox** ____________________

9. **alcohol poisoning** ______________________________

10. **congeners** ______________________________

11. **microsomal ethanol-oxidizing system (MEOS)** ______________________________

◎ Fill-in-the-Blank

1. ______________________________ is a toxic intermediate compound formed by the action of the alcohol dehydrogenase enzyme during the metabolism of alcohol.
2. Inflammation of the stomach is known as ______________________________.
3. The enzyme that catalyzes the conversion of acetaldehyde to acetate ______________________________ ______________________________.
4. Inflammation of the esophagus is called ______________________________.
5. ______________________________ is the enzyme that catalyzes the oxidation of ethanol and other alcohols.
6. The common name for ______________________________, the simplest alcohol, is ______________________________.
7. ______________________________ is the anaerobic conversion of various carbohydrates to carbon dioxide and an alcohol or organic acid.

◎ Fill-in-the-Blank Summaries

Alcohol Metabolism

In the first stage of alcohol metabolism, alcohol dehydrogenase catalyzes the conversion of alcohol to __________. As much as 20% of alcohol is changed to that substance in the __________. The metabolic reactions that convert alcohol to the above consume NAD+ while forming NADH. The resulting build up dramatically slows the citric acid cycle. As a result cells route most of the acetyl CoA to the synthesis of ________.

As alcohol builds up in the body, the body recognizes it as foreign and routes it into the primary overflow pathway called the ________. The ________ ordinarily uses this system to metabolize drugs and detoxify foreign substances. When exposed to large doses of alcohol repeatedly, this pathway's capacity and speed increase.

Alcoholics and Malnutrition

Folate, thiamin and ____________________ are the vitamins most often affected by alcoholism. Thiamin deficiency contributes to the classic conditions of alcoholism such as the brain damage of Wernicke-Korsakoff syndrome. Magnesium deficiency due to alcoholism may cause ____________________. Unless there is bleeding, an alcoholic's __________________ levels tend to be higher than normal in the blood and liver. Copper and ______________________ may be elevated during advanced stages of alcoholism.

Large amounts of alcohol in the blood have the effect of raising __________________ levels. When chronic heavy drinkers eat a normal diet they ____________________.

Notes

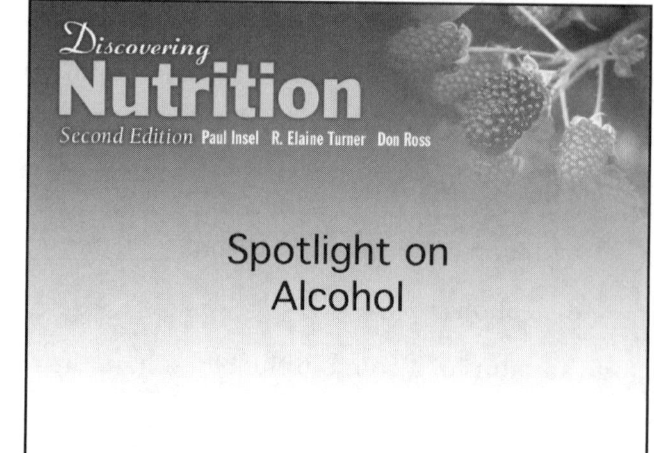

Alcohol

- The character of alcohol
  - Ethanol
    - The alcohol in beer, wine, spirits
  - Methanol
    - Wood alcohol—poisonous
- Is alcohol a nutrient?
  - Provides energy
    - 7 kcal/g
  - No other nutritive value

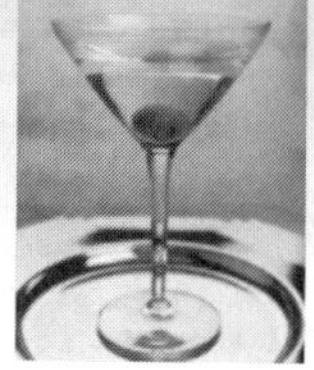

Photos © PhotoDisc

Alcohol and Its Sources

- Fermentation
  - Yeast cells metabolize sugar to make alcohol
- Alcoholic beverages
  - Beer: 5–6% alcohol
  - Wine: 8–14% alcohol
  - Liquor: 35–45% alcohol
    - "Proof" is twice the alcohol percentage

Photo © PhotoDisc

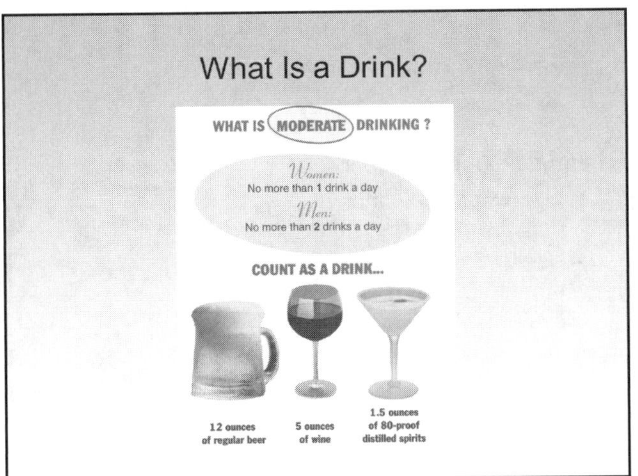

What Is a Drink?
WHAT IS MODERATE DRINKING ?
Women:
No more than 1 drink a day
Men:
No more than 2 drinks a day
COUNT AS A DRINK...
12 ounces of regular beer
5 ounces of wine
1.5 ounces of 80-proof distilled spirits

Alcohol Absorption

- No digestion required
- Absorbed from mouth, esophagus, stomach, and small intestine
- Absorption slowed by food

ALCOHOL ABSORPTION

Small amounts of alcohol are absorbed in the mouth and esophagus

Alcohol is readily absorbed in the stomach, but food will dilute the alcohol and delay gastric emptying

The primary site of alcohol absorption is the upper small intestine

Alcohol Metabolism

- Small amounts of alcohol
  - Alcohol dehydrogenase
    - Alcohol ← acetaldehyde
  - Aldehyde dehydrogenase
    - Acetaldehyde ← acetate
  - Acetaldehyde, acetate converted to acetyl CoA
    - Acetyl CoA molecules built into fatty acids

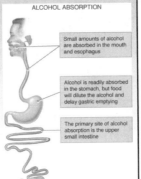

Small amounts of alcohol

Alcohol (ethanol)

Alcohol dehydrogenase

Acetaldehyde

Acetaldehyde dehydrogenase

Citric acid cycle

Acetyl CoA

Little acetyl CoA enters citric acid cycle

Fatty acids

Fat (triglycerides)

Notes

Notes

Alcohol Metabolism

- Large amount of alcohol
  - Overwhelms alcohol dehydrogenase system
  - Uses microsomal ethanol-oxidizing system (MEOS)

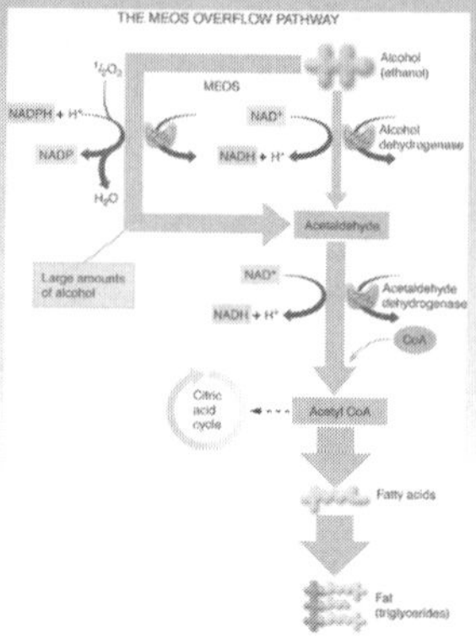

Alcohol Metabolism

- Removing alcohol from circulation
  - Liver metabolism limited
  - Blood alcohol level falls slowly
- Individual differences in rate of alcohol metabolism
  - Gender
  - Race/ethnicity
  - Age

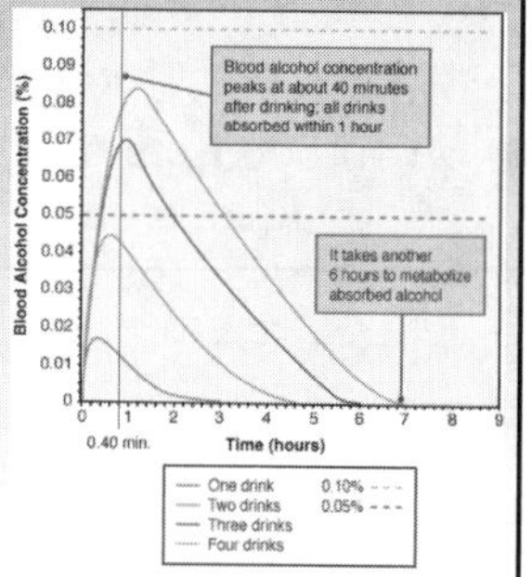

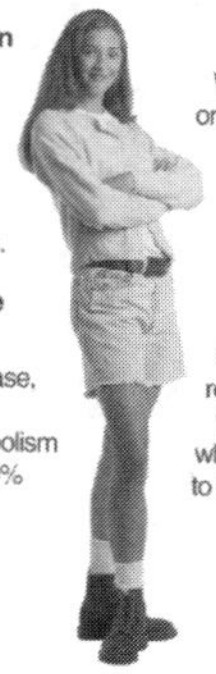

Graph source: National Institute on Alcohol Abuse and Alcoholism

Alcohol Metabolism: Gender Differences

Body composition
Women have a higher percentage of fat than men (size for size women have less water than men to dilute alcohol).

Less enzyme activity
Alcohol dehydrogenase, the primary enzyme involved in the metabolism of alcohol, is up to 40% less active in women than in men.

Body size
Women are smaller on average than men (smaller livers and less total water).

Hormonal fluctuations
Women typically have a heightened response to alcohol which is increased when they are about to have their periods, or when taking birth control pills.

When Alcohol Becomes a Problem

- Alcohol in the brain and nervous system
  - Depressant; affects all parts of brain
- Alcohol's effect on GI system
  - Esophagitis, gastritis

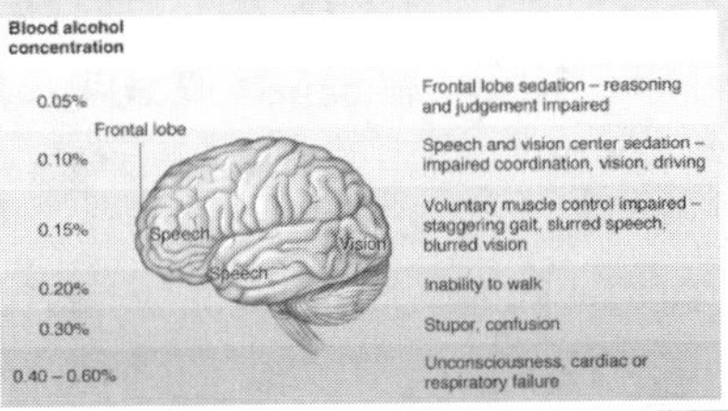

When Alcohol Becomes a Problem

- Alcohol and the liver
  - Fatty liver
  - Fibrosis
  - Cirrhosis
- Fetal alcohol syndrome
  - Physical abnormalities
  - Mental retardation
  - Low birth weight; poor growth

Alcoholics and Malnutrition

- Poor diet
  - Alcohol provides energy but no nutrients
  - Economic factors
  - Lack of interest in food; GI problems
- Vitamin deficiencies
  - Alcohol interferes with vitamin metabolism
  - Folate, thiamin, vitamin A

Poor diet
Vitamin deficiencies
Elevated blood triglycerides
Alcoholism
Mineral deficiencies
Elevated iron, copper, nickel in blood

Notes

Notes

Alcoholics and Malnutrition

- Mineral deficiencies
  - Inadequate diet; fluid losses
  - Calcium, magnesium, iron, zinc
  - Some mineral levels are elevated
- Macronutrients
  - Alcohol interferes with amino acid absorption
  - Alcohol raises blood levels of fats
- Body weight
  - Inconsistent effect of alcohol calories on weight

Does Alcohol Have Benefits?

- Moderate drinking has been associated with reduced mortality
- Heart disease
  - French paradox: red wine

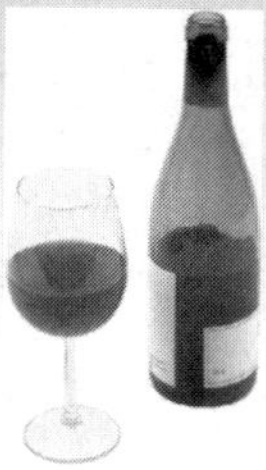

Photo © PhotoDisc

Harmful Effects

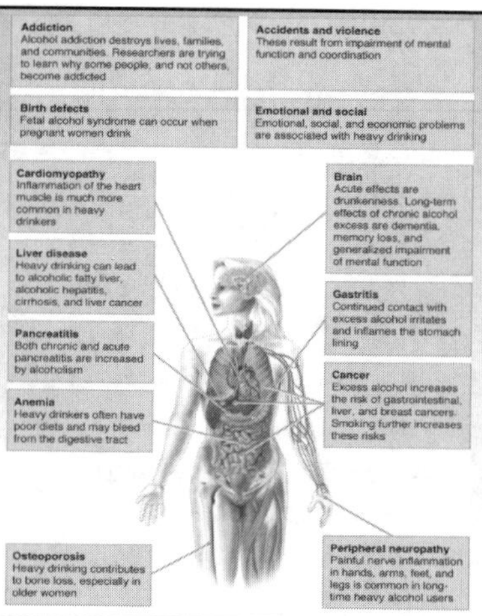

Addiction
Alcohol addiction destroys lives, families, and communities. Researchers are trying to learn why some people, and not others, become addicted

Accidents and violence
These result from impairment of mental function and coordination

Birth defects
Fetal alcohol syndrome can occur when pregnant women drink

Emotional and social
Emotional, social, and economic problems are associated with heavy drinking

Cardiomyopathy
Inflammation of the heart muscle is much more common in heavy drinkers

Brain
Acute effects are drunkenness. Long-term effects of chronic alcohol excess are dementia, memory loss, and generalized impairment of mental function

Liver disease
Heavy drinking can lead to alcoholic fatty liver, alcoholic hepatitis, cirrhosis, and liver cancer

Gastritis
Continued contact with excess alcohol irritates and inflames the stomach lining

Pancreatitis
Both chronic and acute pancreatitis are increased by alcoholism

Cancer
Excess alcohol increases the risk of gastrointestinal, liver, and breast cancers. Smoking further increases these risks

Anemia
Heavy drinkers often have poor diets and may bleed from the digestive tract

Osteoporosis
Heavy drinking contributes to bone loss, especially in older women

Peripheral neuropathy
Painful nerve inflammation in hands, arms, feet, and legs is common in long-time heavy alcohol users

Alcohol

- People who should not consume alcohol
  - Those who cannot moderate intake
  - Children and adolescents
  - Those taking certain medications
  - Those with illnesses worsened by alcohol
  - Those who drive or operate machinery
  - Pregnant or breastfeeding women
  - Those with a strong family history of alcoholism

Notes

CHAPTER 10

Water and Minerals: The Ocean Within

The chapter outline provides you with an organizational guide to the topics and ideas presented in this chapter of the text.

Water: Crucial to Life
- Electrolytes and Water: A Delicate Balance
- Functions of Water

Intake Recommendations: How Much Water Is Enough?
- Water Excretion: Where Does the Water Go?
- Water Balance
- Alcohol, Caffeine, and Common Medications Affect Fluid Balance
- Dehydration
- Water Intoxication

Minerals
- Minerals in Foods
- Bioavailability

Major Minerals and Health
- Hypertension
- Osteoporosis

Sodium
- Dietary Recommendations and Sources of Sodium
- Dealing with Excess Sodium

Potassium
- Dietary Recommendations and Sources of Potassium
- When Potassium Balance Goes Awry

Chloride
- Dietary Recommendations and Sources of Chloride
- Who Risks Chloride Deficiency?

Calcium
- Functions of Calcium
- Regulation of Blood Calcium Levels
- Dietary Recommendations for Calcium
- Sources of Calcium
- Calcium Absorption
- When Calcium Balance Goes Awry

Phosphorus
- Dietary Recommendations and Sources of Phosphorus
- When Phosphate Balance Goes Awry

Magnesium
- Dietary Recommendations and Sources of Magnesium
- When Magnesium Balance Goes Awry

Sulfur

Trace Minerals

Iron
- Functions of Iron
- Regulation of Iron in the Body
- Dietary Recommendations for Iron
- Sources of Iron
- Iron Deficiency
- Iron Toxicity

Zinc
- Functions of Zinc
- Regulation of Zinc in the Body
- Dietary Recommendations for Zinc
- Sources of Zinc
- Zinc Deficiency
- Zinc Toxicity

Key Terms

Define the following terms.

1. **fluorosis** ________________
2. **calmodulin** ________________
3. **ions** ________________
4. **aldosterone** ________________
5. **plasma** ________________
6. **albumin** ________________
7. **osteoblasts** ________________
8. **oxalate (oxalic acid)** ________________
9. **transferrin** ________________
10. **salts** ________________
11. **ceruloplasmin** ________________
12. **hemosiderin** ________________
13. **Lou Gehrig's disease** ________________
14. **ferritin** ________________
15. **insensible water loss** ________________

16. electrolytes ____________

17. diastolic ____________

18. fibrin ____________

19. geophagia ____________

20. essential hypertension ____________

21. Menkes' syndrome ____________

22. hypogonadism ____________

23. osmosis ____________

24. phytate (phytic acid) ____________

25. heme iron ____________

26. systolic ____________

Fill-in-the-Blank

1. ____________ is a hormone secreted by the pituitary gland that increases blood pressure and prevents fluid excretion by the kidneys.

2. ____________ is a genetic disorder of increased copper absorption, which leads to toxic levels in the liver and heart.

3. A hereditary disorder in which excessive absorption of iron results in abnormal iron deposits in the liver and other tissues is ____________.

4. The addition of minerals, such as calcium and phosphate, to bones and teeth is called ____________.

5. ____________ are ions that carry a negative charge, while ____________ are ions that carry a positive charge.

6. Organic compounds that may produce bitterness in coffee and tea are called ____________.

7. ____________ is a congenital condition often caused by severe iodine deficiency during gestation; it is characterized by arrested physical and mental development.

8. ____________ is a selenium-deficiency disease that impairs the structure and function of the heart.

9. A ____________ is a chronic enlargement of the thyroid gland, visible as a swelling at the front of the neck; it is usually associated with iodine deficiency.

10. ______________________________ is the result of a lowered level of circulating thyroid hormone with slowing of mental and physical functions.

11. ______________________________ is a crystalline mineral compound of calcium and phosphorus that makes up bone.

12. A progressive disease that destroys the myelin sheath surrounding nerve fibers of the brain and spinal cord is ______________________________.

13. Compounds that interfere with iodine absorption and can induce goiter are called ______________________________.

14. ______________________________ is a condition in which resting blood pressure persistently exceeds 140 mm Hg systolic or 90 mm Hg diastolic.

15. ______________________________ are present in the body and required in the diet in relatively small amounts compared with major minerals; they are also known as microminerals.

16. Wavelike motion of small hairlike projections on some cells is called ______________________________.

17. The term ______________________________ describes iron or steel with a thin layer of zinc plated onto it to protect against corrosion.

18. A chemical complex with a central iron atom that forms the oxygen-binding part of hemoglobin and myoglobin is ______________________________.

19. The oxygen-transporting protein of muscle that resembles blood hemoglobin in function is ______________________________.

20. The ______________________________ is a hormone secreted from the pituitary gland at the base of the brain that regulates synthesis of thyroid hormones.

21. ______________________________ are bone cells that break down bone structure and release calcium and phosphate into the blood.

22. The iron in plants and animal foods that is not part of hemoglobin or myoglobin is called ______________________________.

23. ______________________________ are required in the diet and present in the body in large amounts compared to trace minerals.

24. Toxicity from excess iron is called ______________________________.

◎ Fill-in-the-Blank Summaries

Water: The Essential Ingredient for Life

Overall, water makes up ____________ percent of your weight. The body maintains its electrolyte balance through the intake and excretion of water and the movement of ions. Positively charged ions are known as ______________________. Negatively charged ions are known as ______________________. About _______________ of body water is in the intracellular fluid, and ____________________ is in extracellular fluid. The major components of extracellular fluid are interstitial fluid and ____________ _______________. To maintain the balance of sodium and potassium, all cell membranes incorporate sodium-potassium pumps that actively pump sodium out of the cell while allowing potassium back in. When electrolytes are more concentrated on one side of the membrane, then ____________________ ________________________________. Cells must contain the right amount of water. Too much and the cell will burst; too little and the cell will shrink. Too much water in the surrounding spaces causes ____.

Minerals

Minerals are essential ______________________________. Absorption of them is limited by several factors, among them ____________________________________ and ____________________________________. Unlike vitamins, minerals are not destroyed by ______________________, ______________________, and _______________________. Like vitamins, however, minerals are "micronutrients." They are needed in relatively ________________________________ amounts. Minerals are often grouped as major minerals and trace minerals. Compared with major minerals, the total amount of trace mineral in your body is _________________________________. Foods from both plants and animals are sources of minerals. Generally speaking, however, ____ are more reliable mineral sources. There are ____________________________ major minerals. Two disorders in which major minerals play critical parts are hypertension and _________________________, which primarily affects ________________________________.

Notes

Discovering
Nutrition
Second Edition Paul Insel R. Elaine Turner Don Ross

Water and Minerals:
The Ocean Within

Chapter 10

Water: Crucial to Life

- Water is the most essential nutrient
- Electrolytes and water
  - Balanced inside and outside cells

Functions of Water

Resistance to temperature change (heat capacity)
Cooling
FUNCTIONS OF WATER
Body fluids
pH balance
Chemical reactions

Water Balance

- Fluid input
  - Beverages
  - Foods
  - Metabolism
- Fluid output
  - Kidneys
  - Skin
  - Lungs
  - Feces

Regulation of Water Balance

- Hormonal effects
  - Antidiuretic hormone (ADH)
  - Aldosterone
- Thirst
- Substances that affect water balance
  - Alcohol and diuretic medications

Understanding Minerals

- Minerals
  - Inorganic elements
  - Involved in body structure, regulation
  - Found in plant and animal foods
  - Major minerals and trace minerals

Notes

Notes

Major Minerals and Health

- Hypertension: high blood pressure
  - Increases risk for heart disease, stroke, kidney disease
  - Risk factors for hypertension
    - Obesity
    - High sodium intake
    - Lack of physical activity
    - Excess alcohol intake
    - Race
    - Age
    - Family history

Major Minerals and Health

- Sodium and hypertension
  - Reducing sodium intake lowers blood pressure (BP)
- Other dietary factors
  - High chloride intake increases BP
  - High calcium, magnesium, and potassium intake lowers BP

Major Minerals and Health

- Osteoporosis
  - Decreased bone density
  - Develops gradually with age
  - Women at higher risk
  - Adequate calcium intake reduces risk

Major Minerals and Health

- Osteoporosis
  - Factors to reduce risk
    - Diet rich in calcium and vitamin D
    - Regular physical activity
    - Healthy body weight
    - Minimize chances of falling
    - Avoid smoking and excess alcohol intake

Sodium

- Functions
  - Fluid balance
  - Nerve impulse transmission
- Food sources
  - Salt
  - Processed and convenience foods

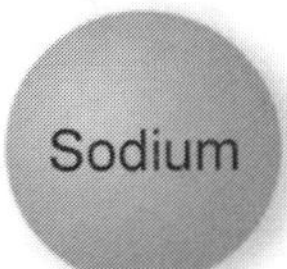

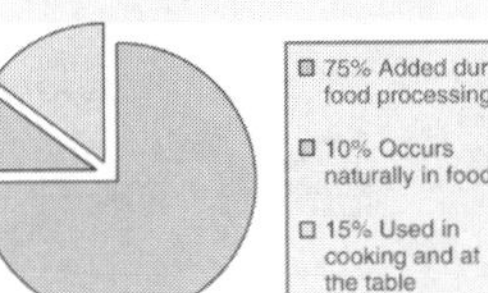

Potassium

- Functions
  - Muscle contraction
  - Nerve impulse transmission
  - Fluid balance
- Food sources
  - Unprocessed foods: fruits, vegetables, grains

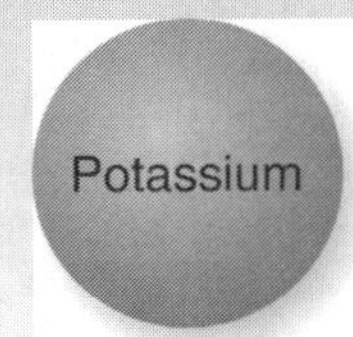

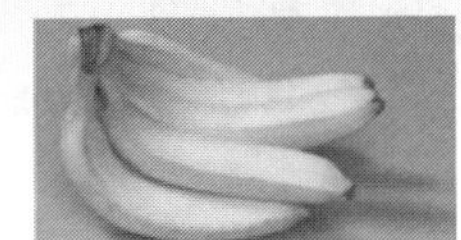

Photo © PhotoDisc

Notes

Notes

Chloride

- Functions of chloride
  - Fluid balance
  - Hydrochloric acid (stomach acid)
- Food sources of chloride
  - Table salt

Chloride

Calcium

- Functions
  - Bone structure
  - Blood clotting
  - Nerve impulse transmission, muscle contraction
- Food sources
  - Milk and dairy products
  - Green vegetables, tofu, fortified foods

Calcium

Photo@DigitalStock

Phosphorus

- Functions
  - Bone structure
  - Component of ATP, DNA, RNA, phospholipids
- Food sources
  - Meat, milk, eggs
  - Processed foods

Phosphorus

Photo@Photodisc

Notes

Iron

Iron

- Functions
  - Oxygen transport as part of hemoglobin and myoglobin
  - Cofactor for enzymes, normal brain and immune function
- Food sources
  - Red meats, liver, seafood

Iron

- Deficiency
  - Iron-deficiency anemia
- Toxicity
  - Poisoning in children
  - Hemochromatosis

Normal cells
Decrease in iron stores
Decrease in iron transport
Development of iron deficiency
Fall in hemoglobin synthesis leads to anemia
Anemic cells

Zinc

Zinc

- Functions
  - Cofactor for enzymes
  - Gene regulation, immune health
- Food sources
  - Red meats, seafood
- Deficiency
  - Poor growth, delayed development
- Toxicity
  - Can cause copper deficiency

Photo@Photodisc

Notes

Selenium

- Functions
  - Part of antioxidant enzyme
  - Thyroid metabolism, immune function
- Food sources
  - Organ meats, fish, seafood, meats, Brazil nuts

Selenium

Selenium

- Deficiency
  - Increases susceptibility to some infections
- Toxicity
  - Brittle hair and nails

Iodine

- Functions
  - Thyroid hormone production
- Food sources
  - Iodized salt, fish, seafood, dairy products

Iodine

Photo@Photodisc

Iodine

- Deficiency
  - Goiter: enlarged thyroid gland
  - Cretinism: mental retardation
    - Occurs in fetus when pregnant woman is deficient

Copper

- Functions of copper
  - Melanin, collagen, elastin production
  - Immune function
  - Antioxidant enzyme systems
- Food sources of copper
  - Organ meats, shellfish, nuts, legumes

Copper

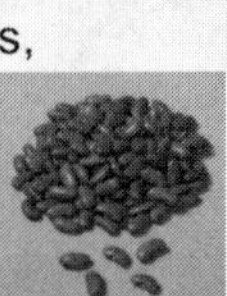

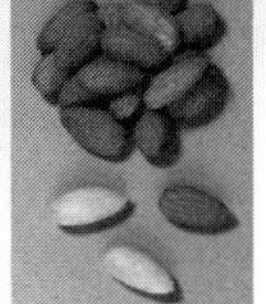

Photos@Digital Stock

Manganese

- Functions of manganese
  - Cartilage production
  - Antioxidant enzyme systems
- Food sources of manganese
  - Tea, coffee, nuts, cereals

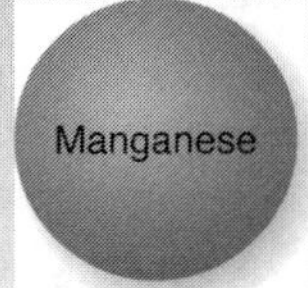

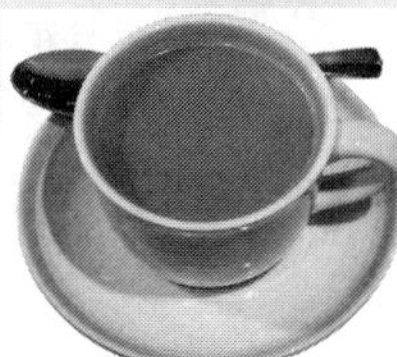

Photo@LiquidLibrary

Notes

Notes

Fluoride

- Functions
  - Bone and tooth structure
- Food sources
  - Fluoridated water
- Fluoride balance
  - Excess can cause fluorosis

Fluoride

Chromium

- Functions
  - Glucose metabolism
- Food sources
  - Mushrooms, dark chocolate, nuts, whole grains

Chromium

Photo@Digital Stock

Molybdenum

- Functions
  - Enzyme cofactor
- Food sources
  - Peas, beans, some breakfast cereals, organ meats

CHAPTER 11

Sports Nutrition: Eating for Peak Performance

The chapter outline provides you with an organizational guide to the topics and ideas presented in this chapter of the text.

Nutrition and Physical Performance
Energy Systems, Muscles, and Physical Performance
- ATP-CP Energy System
- Lactic Acid Energy System
- Oxygen Energy System
- Teamwork in Energy Production
- Glycogen Depletion
- Endurance Training
- Muscles and Muscle Fibers

Optimal Nutrition for Athletic Performance
Energy Intake and Exercise
Carbohydrate and Exercise
- Carbohydrate Loading
- Carbohydrate Intake Before Exercise
- Carbohydrate Intake During Exercise
- Carbohydrate Intake Following Exercise

Dietary Fat and Exercise
- Fat Intake and the Athlete

Protein and Exercise
- Protein Recommendations for Athletes
- Protein Intake and the Athlete
- Protein Intake After Exercise
- Dangers of High Protein Intake

Vitamins, Minerals, and Athletic Performance
- B Vitamins
- Calcium
- Iron
- Other Trace Minerals

Fluid Needs during Exercise
- Hydration: Drink More!

Nutrition Needs of Youth in Sport
Nutrition Supplements and Ergogenic Aids
- Amino Acids
- "Andro" and DHEA
- Caffeine
- Carnitine
- Chromium
- Coenzyme Q_{10} (Ubiquinone)
- Colostrum
- Creatine
- Ephedrine
- Ginseng
- Glutamine
- Medium-Chain Triglyceride Oil
- Pyruvate
- Ribose
- Sodium Bicarbonate

Weight and Body Composition
- Weight Gain: Build Muscle, Lose Fat
- Weight Loss: The Panacea for Optimal Performance?
- Weight Loss: Negative Consequences for the Competitive Athlete?
- Female Athlete Triad

◎ Key Terms

Define the following terms.

1. **amenorrhea** ______________________________
2. **soda loading** ______________________________
3. **diuresis** ______________________________
4. **creatine** ______________________________
5. **female athlete triad** ______________________________
6. **palatable** ______________________________
7. **slow-twitch (ST) fibers** ______________________________
8. **lactic acid energy system** ______________________________
9. **androstenedione** ______________________________
10. **carbohydrate loading** ______________________________
11. **anabolic steroids** ______________________________
12. **ginseng** ______________________________
13. **aerobic endurance** ______________________________
14. **pathogenic** ______________________________
15. **perceived exertion** ______________________________

◎ Fill-in-the-Blank

1. The ______________________________ is a simple and immediate anaerobic energy system that maintains ATP levels.
2. ______________________________ are muscle fibers that can develop high tension rapidly. These fibers can fatigue quickly, but are well suited to explosive movements in sprinting, jumping, and weight lifting.
3. ______________________________ are muscles composed of bundles of parallel, striated muscle fibers under voluntary control.
4. ______________________________ involves a lowered concentration of hemoglobin in the blood due to dilution.
5. ______________________________ is a steroid that is the precursor to androstenedione. It is secreted primarily by the adrenal gland, but also by the testes.
6. To release ATP, the ______________________________ completes the breakdown of carbohydrate and fatty acids via the citric acid cycle and electron transport chain.

7. ______________________________ is a compound abundant in cells and vital to the production of ATP in the electron transport chain; it is also called ubiquinone.

8. Individual muscle cells are called ______________________________.

9. An energy-rich compound that supplies energy and a phosphate group for the formation of ATP is ______________________________.

10. Substances that can enhance athletic performance are ______________________________.

11. The amount of blood expelled by the heart is ______________________________.

12. ______________________________ occurs when a person has a much higher than normal body temperature.

Fill-in-the-Blank Summaries

Energy for Optimal Performance

Our muscles process fuel in the form of chemical energy to produce power for physical performance. Although your body contains hundreds of muscles, there are only three types of muscles. The ______________________________ muscles are bundles of parallel, striated fibers attached to your skeleton and are under conscious control. There are two types of muscle fibers that make up muscle cells—fast twitch and slow twitch. Slow twitch fibers can maintain muscular activity for a prolonged period. During shorter, higher intensity endurance events like a mile run or a 400-meter swim the body utilizes ______________________________ fibers. ______________________________ determine an individual's percentage of slow twitch fibers and fast twitch fibers.

ATP supplies the energy for muscle fiber contraction and relaxation. To produce ATP your muscles use the ATP–CP energy system, lactic acid energy system, and the oxygen energy system. Muscles store enough ATP to sustain muscle movements for less than a second. The body also stores creatine phosphate, which your muscles can convert to ATP. After 3 to 15 seconds your body has used up its entire ATP and CP stores. Using the anaerobic glycolysis system, also known as the ______________________________, muscle cells can break down thousands of glucose molecules from stored muscle glycogen to form ATP. In comparison to the ATP–CP and the lactic acid energy system, the oxygen energy system produces a low amount of ATP at a fast rate.

Nutrition Supplements and Ergogenic Aids

For most athletes who select a variety of foods and meet their energy needs, supplements are not necessary. ______________________________ supplements are sometimes recommended for female athletes who may not get enough in their diets. The ______________________________ synthesizes the testosterone precursors androstenedione and dehydroepiandrosterone (DHEA). Some claim that supplements of these two precursors will lead to increased testosterone levels and enhanced muscle mass. Researchers have found, however, that the supplements only raise testosterone levels in men. Ginseng has become popular among athletes because reports suggest that it ______________ ________. Several well-controlled studies have shown improvements in muscle strength when ______________________________ supplementation was added to a strength-training regimen, but creatine supplements appear to have no benefit for aerobic training. In the mitochondria of muscle cells, ______________________ actively helps transfer electrons in the electron transport chain.

Notes

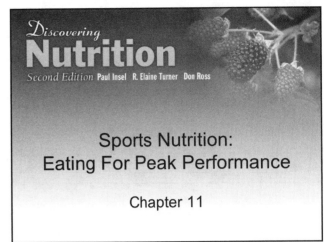
Discovering
Nutrition
Second Edition Paul Insel R. Elaine Turner Don Ross
Sports Nutrition:
Eating For Peak Performance
Chapter 11

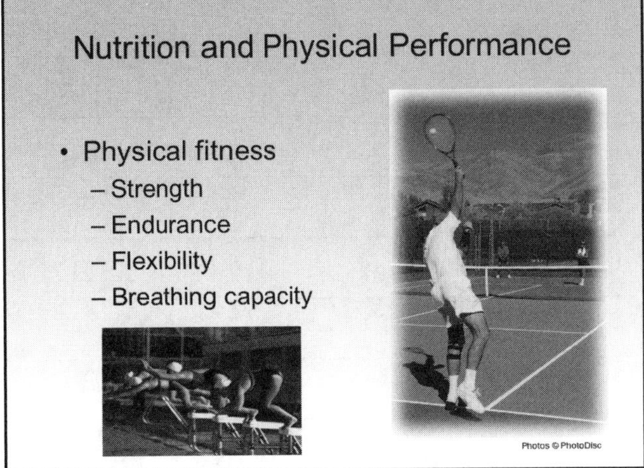
Nutrition and Physical Performance
• Physical fitness
– Strength
– Endurance
– Flexibility
– Breathing capacity
Photos © PhotoDisc

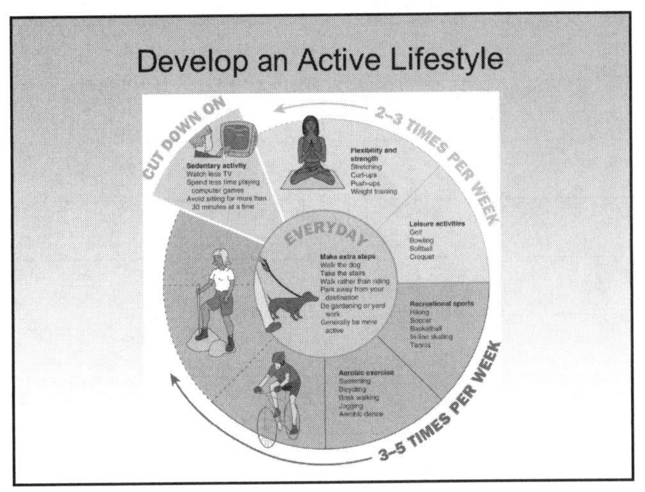
Develop an Active Lifestyle
CUT DOWN ON
Sedentary activity
Watch less TV
Spend less time playing computer games
Avoid sitting for more than 30 minutes at a time
2–3 TIMES PER WEEK
Flexibility and strength
Stretching
Curl-ups
Push-ups
Weight training
Leisure activities
Golf
Bowling
Softball
Croquet
EVERYDAY
Make extra steps
Walk the dog
Take the stairs
Walk rather than riding
Park away from your destination
Do gardening or yard work
Generally be more active
Recreational sports
Hiking
Soccer
Basketball
In-line skating
Tennis
Aerobic exercise
Swimming
Bicycling
Brisk walking
Jogging
Aerobic dance
3–5 TIMES PER WEEK

Notes

Energy Systems, Muscles, and Physical Performance

- ATP-CP energy system
  - Quick source of ATP
    - Cellular ATP and creatine phosphate
  - Fuel for 3 to 15 seconds of maximal effort

Energy Systems for Physical Performance

- Lactic acid energy system
  - Breakdown of glucose to lactic acid (lactate)
    - Doesn't require oxygen
  - Rise in acidity triggers muscle fatigue

Energy Systems, Muscles, and Physical Performance

- Oxygen energy system
  - Breakdown of carbohydrate and fat for energy
    - Requires oxygen
    - Produces ATP more slowly

Energy Systems, Muscles, and Physical Performance

- Teamwork in energy production
  - Anaerobic systems: short-duration activities, early part of endurance activities
  - Aerobic systems: endurance activities
- Training
  - Decreases reliance on anaerobic systems
  - Extends availability of glycogen

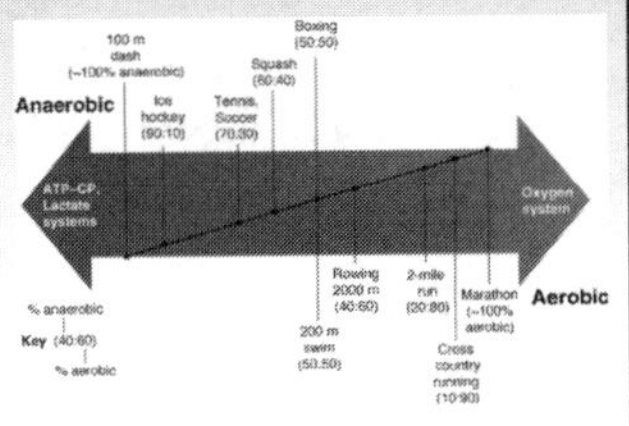

Energy Systems, Muscles, and Physical Performance

- Muscles and muscle fibers
  - Slow-twitch fibers
  - Fast-twitch fibers
    - Relative proportion determined by genetics

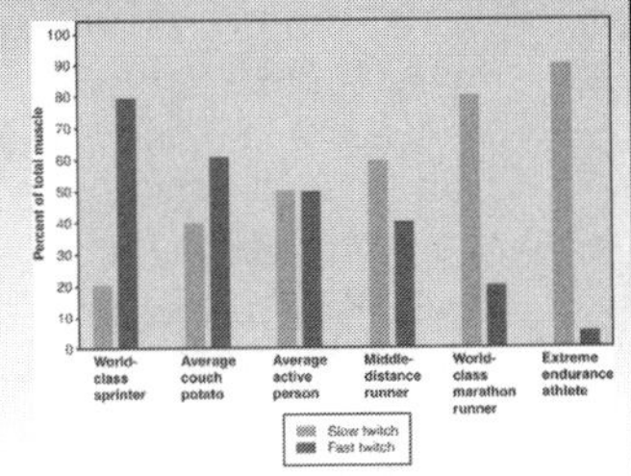

Optimal Nutrition for Athletic Performance

- Consume adequate energy and nutrients
- Maintain appropriate body composition
- Promote optimal recovery from training
- Maintain hydration status

Notes

Notes

Energy Intake and Exercise

- Energy needs
  - Fuel for training
  - Maintain healthy weight
  - Support growth (if adolescent)
  - May require frequent meals and snacks

Carbohydrate and Exercise

- High-carbohydrate diets
  - Increase glycogen stores
  - Extend endurance
- Carbohydrate loading
  - 60–70% of calories as carbohydrate
  - Decrease exercise intensity prior to competition

Carbohydrate and Exercise

- Carbohydrate intake
  - Before exercise
    - Easily digested foods/beverages
  - During exercise
    - Sports drinks (4–8% carbohydrate)
  - After exercise
    - Replenish glycogen stores
      - 1 to 1.5 grams carbohydrate per kg both 30 minutes and 2 hours after exercise

Dietary Fat and Exercise

- Fat
  - Major fuel source for endurance activities
  - High-fat diet not needed
  - Recommendations
    - Moderate fat intake: 20–35% of calories

Protein and Exercise

- Protein recommendations
  - Adults: 0.8 grams per kg body weight
  - Endurance athletes: 1.2–1.4 g/kg
  - Strength athletes: 1.6–1.7 g/kg
- Protein sources
  - Foods: lean meats, fish, low-fat dairy, egg whites
- Protein intake after exercise
  - Helps replenish glycogen
- Dangers of high protein intake

Vitamins, Minerals, and Athletic Performance

- B vitamins
  - Needed for energy metabolism
  - Choose variety of whole grains, fruits, vegetables
- Calcium
  - Needed for normal muscle function, strong bones
  - Low-fat dairy products
  - Adequate intake may be a problem for females

Notes

Notes

Vitamins, Minerals, and Athletic Performance

- Iron
  - Needed for oxygen delivery and energy production
  - Athletes have higher losses
  - Lean red meats, vegetables, enriched grains
- Other trace minerals
  - Copper, zinc
  - Avoid high-dose supplements

Fluid Needs During Exercise

- Exercise and fluid loss
  - Increased losses from sweat
  - Increased with heat, humidity
  - Risk for dehydration

Fluid Needs During Exercise

- Hydration
  - Adequate fluids before, during, after exercise
  - Water vs. sports drinks
    - Duration
    - Intensity
    - Environmental factors

Nutrition Supplements and Ergogenic Aids

- Many product claims
  - Provide energy, enhance performance, change body composition
- Limited scientific evidence
- Potential for side effects
- Many substances are banned for athletes

Weight and Body Composition

- Weight gain
  - Increase muscle, reduce fat
- Weight loss
  - Lose fat, maintain muscle
  - Avoid dangerous weight-loss practices
- Female athlete triad
  - Disordered eating
  - Amenorrhea
  - Osteoporosis

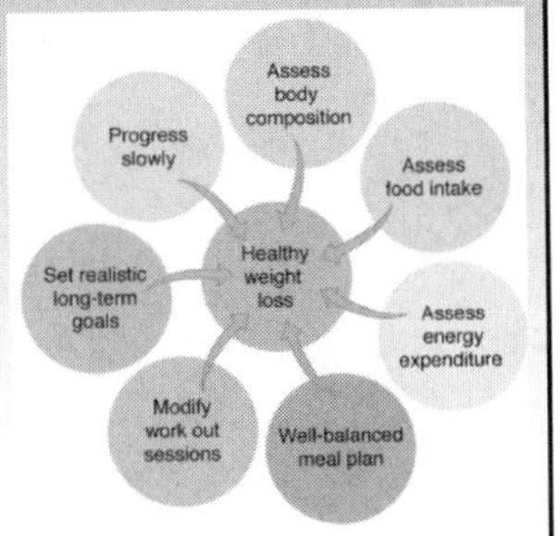

Assess body composition
Assess food intake
Assess energy expenditure
Well-balanced meal plan
Modify work out sessions
Set realistic long-term goals
Progress slowly
Healthy weight loss

Notes

SPOTLIGHT ON

Eating Disorders

The Spotlight outline provides you with an organizational guide to the topics and ideas presented in this section of the text.

The Eating Disorder Continuum
History of a Modern Malady
No Simple Causes
Anorexia Nervosa
- Causes of Anorexia Nervosa
- Warning Signs
- Treatment

Bulimia Nervosa
- Causes of Bulimia
- Obsessed by Thoughts of Food
- Treatment

Binge-Eating Disorder
- Stress and Conflict Often Trigger Binge Eating
- Treatment

Body Dysmorphic Disorder
Night-Eating Syndrome
Males: An Overlooked Population
- An Unrecognized Disorder

Anorexia Athletica
The Female Athlete Triad
Vegetarianism and Eating Disorders
Smoking and Eating Disorders
Baryophobia
Infantile Anorexia
Combating Eating Disorders

◎ Key Terms

Define the following terms.

1. **eating disorders** ______________________________
2. **body image** ______________________________
3. **emetics** ______________________________
4. **laxatives** ______________________________
5. **purge** ______________________________
6. **disordered eating** ______________________________
7. **enemas** ______________________________

8. night-eating syndrome (NES) ____________________

9. orexin ____________________

10. infantile anorexia ____________________

11. binge ____________________

◎ Fill-in-the-Blank

1. ____________________ is an eating disorder marked by repeated episodes of binge eating and a feeling of loss of control. A person with this disorder does not follow binge eating with self-induced vomiting or other such practices. The diagnosis is based on a person's having an average of at least two binge-eating episodes per week for six months.

2. ____________________ is an eating disorder marked by prolonged decrease of appetite and refusal to eat, leading to self-starvation and excessive weight loss. It results in part from a distorted body image and intense fear of becoming fat, often linked to social pressures.

3. Drugs or other substances that promote the formation and release of urine are ____________________. They are given to reduce body fluid volume in treating such disorders as high blood pressure, congestive heart disease, and edema.

4. An anxiety disorder characterized by an emotional response to a traumatic event or situation involving severe external stress is called ____________________.

5. ____________________ is an eating disorder associated with competitive participation in athletic activity.

6. ____________________ is an uncommon eating disorder that stunts growth in children and young adults as a result of underfeeding.

7. ____________________ is an eating disorder in which a distressing and impairing preoccupation with an imagined or slight defect in appearance is the primary symptom.

8. ____________________ is an eating disorder marked by consumption of large amounts of food at one time followed by a behavior such as self-induced vomiting, use of laxatives, excessive exercise, fasting, or other practices to avoid weight gain.

◎ Fill-in-the-Blank Summaries

Anorexia

Until the ______________________________, anorexia nervosa was a relatively obscure disease. Today an estimated ______________________________ females between the ages of 13 and 19 suffer from anorexia. Those who suffer from anorexia are obsessed with ______________________________ but are more obsessed with ______________________________. Because most cases of anorexia begin during puberty, some experts believe that it may be related to ______________________________. Most experts agree that anorexia cannot ever be completely cured and that patients will struggle somewhat for the rest of their lives. The earlier the person receives treatment, the better the prognosis. The first goal of treatment is to ______________________________. ______________________________, ______________________________, and ______________________________ are often necessary for treatment.

Bulimia Nervosa

Bulimia nervosa has been recognized as an eating disorder since ______________________. Bulimic patients are usually in their twenties or thirties and tend to feel ________________. To meet the official DSM-IV definition of the disorder, bingeing and purging must occur at least ______________________________. Bulimic patients who frequently purge develop a variety of physical symptoms such as ______________________________. The body weight of people with bulimia is typically ______________________________. During treatment for bulimia nervosa, patients may also be treated for substance abuse and ______________________________.

Notes

Discovering Nutrition
Second Edition Paul Insel R. Elaine Turner Don Ross

Spotlight on Eating Disorders

Eating Disorders

- Eating disorders vs. disordered eating
- The eating disorder continuum

Anorexia Nervosa — Bulimia Nervosa — Binge-eating disorder
self-starvation — binge & purge — compulsive overeating

Eating Disorders: No Simple Causes

- Predisposition
- Social factors
  - Expectations for body size, shape
- Psychological factors
  - Peer relationships
  - Family expectations
  - Emotional trauma
- Biological factors
  - Neurotransmitter levels
- Genetic factors
  - Synthesis and release of leptin, orexin

Anorexia Nervosa

- Diagnostic criteria
  - Body weight < 85% of expected (BMI £ 17.5 kg/m^2)
  - Intense fear of weight gain
  - Distorted body image
  - Amenorrhea
- Causes
- Warning signs

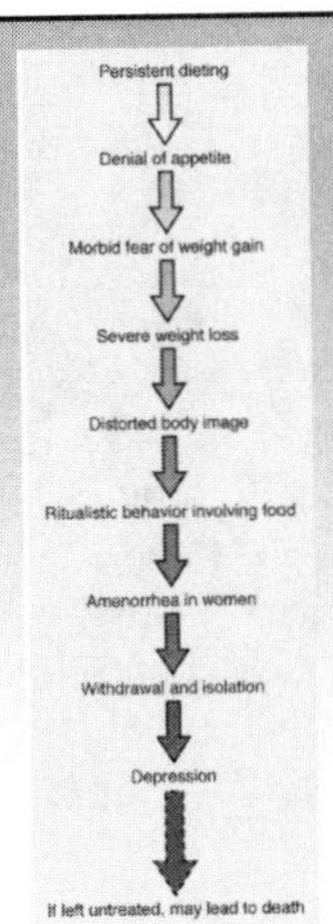

Anorexia Nervosa: Treatment

- Goals
  - Stabilize physical condition
  - Convert patient into participant
  - Restore nutritional status
  - Gradual weight gain
- Psychotherapy
  - Individual
  - Group
  - Family

Bulimia Nervosa

- Diagnostic criteria
  - Recurrent binge eating
  - Recurrent purging, excessive exercise, fasting
  - Excessive concern about weight, shape
  - Absence of anorexia nervosa
- Causes

Notes

Notes

Bulimia Nervosa: Binge/Purge Cycle

- Binge: large amount of food, short period of time
  - High-calorie, high- fat foods
- Purge
  - Affects fluid and electrolyte balance
  - Can be life threatening

Bulimia Nervosa: Treatment

- Medical
- Nutritional
- Psychotherapy
  - Antidepressant medications

Binge-Eating Disorder

- Diagnostic criteria
  - Recurrent binge eating
  - Distress over eating behaviors
  - No recurrent purging
  - Absence of anorexia nervosa
- Triggers of binge eating
  - Stress
  - Conflict
  - Frequent dieting

Binge-Eating Disorder: Treatment

- Psychotherapy
  - Antidepressant medications
- Long-term support

Loneliness
Depression
Anxiety
Stress

Eating Disorders: Other Issues

- Other related conditions
  - Body dysmorphic disorder
  - Night-eating syndrome
- Males: an overlooked population
  - Fewer instances than females
  - Men involved in sports, modeling, entertainment
    - Pressure for certain weight, shape
- Anorexia athletica
  - Sports-related eating disorders
  - Body size/shape important in competition
  - Pressure from coaches

Eating Disorders: Other Issues

- Female athlete triad
  - Disordered eating
  - Amenorrhea
  - Osteoporosis

Disordered Eating
Amenorrhea
Osteoporosis

Notes

Notes

Eating Disorders: Other Issues

- Vegetarianism and eating disorders
- Smoking and eating disorders
- Baryophobia
- Infantile anorexia

Preventing Eating Disorders

- Promote self-esteem
- Size acceptance
- Celebrate the diversity in all sizes and shapes
- Discourage meal skipping
- Encourage eating in response to hunger, not emotions

CHAPTER 12

Life Cycle: Maternal and Infant Nutrition

The chapter outline provides you with an organizational guide to the topics and ideas presented in this chapter of the text.

◎ Key Terms

Define the following terms.

1. **colostrum** ______________________________
2. **infancy** ______________________________
3. **extrusion reflex** ______________________________
4. **amniotic fluid** ______________________________
5. **growth charts** ______________________________
6. **organogenesis** ______________________________
7. **critical period of development** ______________________________
8. **let-down reflex** ______________________________

9. **lactation** ______________________________

10. **neonate** ______________________________

11. **colic** ______________________________

12. **full-term baby** ______________________________

13. **failure to thrive (FTT)** ______________________________

14. **gestational diabetes** ______________________________

15. **low-birth-weight infant** ______________________________

16. **preeclampsia** ______________________________

Fill-in-the-Blanks

1. The first stage of gestation, during which tissue proliferation by rapid cell division begins, is the ______________________________.

2. The ______________________________ is a USDA program that provides federal grants to states for supplemental foods, health care referrals, and nutrition education for low-income pregnant, breastfeeding, and nonbreastfeeding postpartum women and to infants and children at nutritional risk.

3. The developmental stage between the time of implantation (about two weeks after fertilization) through the seventh or eighth week is called the ______________________________.

4. A backflow of stomach contents into the esophagus, accompanied by a burning pain because of the acidity of the gastric juices is called ______________________________.

5. A delivery that occurs before the 37th week of gestation is a ______________________________.

6. ______________________________ is a pituitary hormone that stimulates the release of milk from the breast.

7. ______________________________ are the three equal time periods of pregnancy, each lasting approximately 13 to 14 weeks.

8. Any foods or liquids other than breast milk or infant formula fed to an infant are ______________________________.

9. The period of rapid growth from the end of the embryonic stage until birth is the ______________________________.

10. Health professionals trained to specialize in education about and promotion of breastfeeding are known as ______________________.

11. The measurement of the largest part of the infant's head (just above the eyebrow and ears) is ______________________; this is used to determine brain growth.

12. ______________________ is a pituitary hormone that stimulates the production of milk in the breast tissue.

13. A child between 12 and 36 months of age is a ______________________.

14. The ______________________ is the organ formed during pregnancy that produces hormones for the maintenance of pregnancy and across which oxygen and nutrients are transferred from mother to infant; it also allows waste materials to be transferred from infant to mother.

15. ______________________ is a persistent or recurring nausea that often occurs in the morning during early pregnancy.

◎ Fill-in-the-Blank Summaries

Pregnancy

Many women choose to have preconception care. Nutrition is part of all three components of preconception care. When a woman takes a folic acid supplement to reduce her baby's chance of having a neural tube defect, she is participating in the component of preconception known as ______________________. Obesity during pregnancy poses a risk of ______________________. A woman who is obese and pregnant should not ______________________. Women should increase their intake of most vitamins and minerals during pregnancy; however, ______________________ can be teratogenic when taken in large amounts, causing birth defects of the head, heart, brain, or spinal cord. Women are advised to avoid consuming more than 100% of the RDA for this nutrient. For women of normal weight, doctors usually recommend that they gain ______________________ pounds during pregnancy. Women who have a BMI of 29 kg/m^2 or greater should gain at least ______________________ pounds. Women need about ______________________ more kilocalories a day during pregnancy. The Institute of Medicine's Nutrient Supplement Subcommittee recommends that during pregnancy women take supplements of ______________________ and ______________________

__________. Experts recommend that during pregnancy women do not consume __________________________ ______________________________.

Lactation

Nearly all women can breastfeed. The final stages in breast tissue that make milk production possible occur ____. During the first two or three days after birth, an infant receives immature milk that is high in protein and immunoglobins called ____. The ____ is the reflex that allows milk to flow from the breast. It is initiated when the infant begins sucking on the breast, but can also be stimulated by hearing the baby cry or thinking about the baby.

For the infant, breastfeeding has been shown to reduce the risk of ____________________________, __________ _______________________, and _______________________________ infections. For a mother, breastfeeding may reduce her disease risk. Breastfeeding also stimulates ____________________________________, which can help control blood loss.

Notes

Discovering Nutrition

Second Edition Paul Insel R. Elaine Turner Don Ross

Life Cycle: Maternal and Infant Nutrition

Chapter 12

Pregnancy

- Nutrition before conception
  - Risk assessment, health promotion, intervention
  - Weight
    - Maintain a healthy weight
    - Low or high weight increases risk for poor outcome

Photo © PhotoDisc

Nutrition Before Conception

- Vitamins
  - 400 micrograms folic acid per day
  - Avoid high doses of vitamin A (retinol)
- Substance use
  - Eliminate prior to pregnancy

Notes

Physiology of Pregnancy

- Stages of human fetal growth
  - Blastogenic stage: first 2 weeks
    - Cells differentiate into fetus, placenta
  - Embryonic stage: weeks 2 to 8
    - Development of organ systems
  - Fetal stage: week 9 to delivery
    - Growth

Physiology of Pregnancy

- Maternal changes
  - Growth of adipose, breast, uterine tissues
  - Increase blood volume
  - Slower GI motility

Maternal Weight Gain

- Recommendations depend on BMI
  - Normal weight (BMI = 19.8 – 26 kg/m^2)
    - Gain 25 to 35 pounds
  - Higher recommended gain for underweight women, teens, multiple fetuses
  - Lower recommended gain for overweight and obese women

Energy and Nutrition During Pregnancy

- Energy
  - Support adequate weight gain
- Macronutrients
  - High carbohydrate, moderate fat and protein
- Micronutrients
  - Increased need for most vitamins and minerals
  - Highest increase for iron and folate

Food Choices for Pregnant Women

- Follow MyPyramid
- Supplements of iron and folate
- Foods to avoid
  - Alcohol
  - Certain types of fish

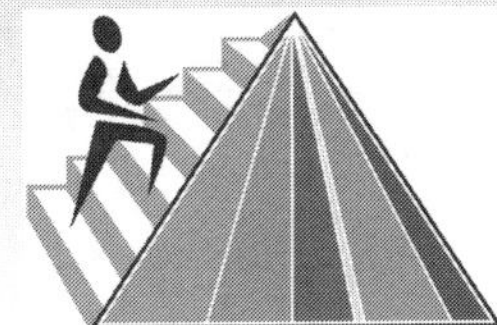

Substance Use and Pregnancy Outcome

- Tobacco
  - Risk for miscarriage, stillbirth, preterm delivery, low birth weight
- Alcohol
  - Risk for fetal alcohol syndrome
    - Physical and mental defects
    - Growth retardation
- Drugs
  - Risks for low birth weight, preterm delivery, miscarriage, birth defects, infant addiction

Notes

Notes

Special Situations During Pregnancy: GI Distress

Avoiding GI distress

Reduce morning sickness
- Eat dry cereal, toast, or crackers before getting out of bed

Reduce constipation
- Eat/drink plenty of fiber and fluids
- Get regular, moderate exercise

Reduce heartburn
- Remain upright for an hour after eating
- Eat smaller amounts more frequently

Special Situations During Pregnancy

- Food cravings and aversions
- Hypertension
- Diabetes
- Gestational diabetes
- AIDS
- Adolescence

Lactation

- Breastfeeding trends
- Healthy People 2010 goals
  - 75% of infants breastfed initially
  - 50% of infants still breastfed at 6 months

Physiology of Lactation

- Changes during adolescence and pregnancy
  - Increased breast tissue
  - Maturation of structure
- After delivery
  - Milk production and secretion
    - Colostrum: first milk

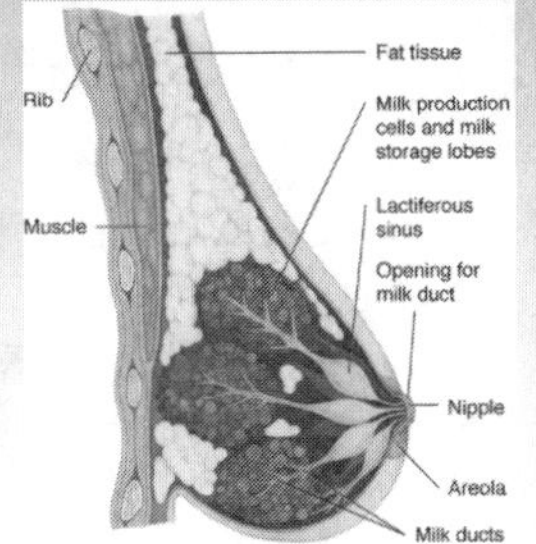

Physiology of Lactation

- Hormonal controls
  - Prolactin: stimulates milk production
  - Oxytocin: stimulates milk release
    - "let-down" reflex

Nutrition for Breastfeeding Women

- Energy and protein
  - Higher needs than during pregnancy
- Vitamins and minerals
  - Most are higher or same as during pregnancy
  - Iron and folate needs are lower
- Water
- Food choices: MyPyramid
- Practices to avoid while breastfeeding
  - Alcohol, drugs, smoking, excess caffeine

Notes

Notes

Benefits of Breastfeeding

- Benefits for infants
  - Optimal nutrition
  - Reduced incidence of respiratory, GI, and ear infections
  - Convenience
  - Other benefits
- Benefits for mother
  - Convenience
  - Enhanced recovery of uterus size
  - Other benefits
- Contraindications to breastfeeding

Infancy

- Growth is the best marker of nutritional status
  - Evaluated using growth charts
- Weight gain
  - Double birth weight by 4 to 6 months
  - Triple birth weight by 12 months
- Length gain
  - Increase length by 50% by 12 months
- Head circumference

Energy and Nutrient Needs During Infancy

- Requirements based on composition of breast milk
  - Energy
    - Highest needs of any life stage
  - Protein
    - Highest needs of any life stage
  - Carbohydrate and fat
    - Fat: major energy source
    - Carbohydrates as simple sugars
  - Water

Energy and Nutrient Needs During Infancy

- Key vitamins and minerals
  - Vitamin D
  - Vitamin K
  - Vitamin B_{12}
  - Iron
  - Fluoride
- Feeding infants
  - Breast milk
  - Infant formula

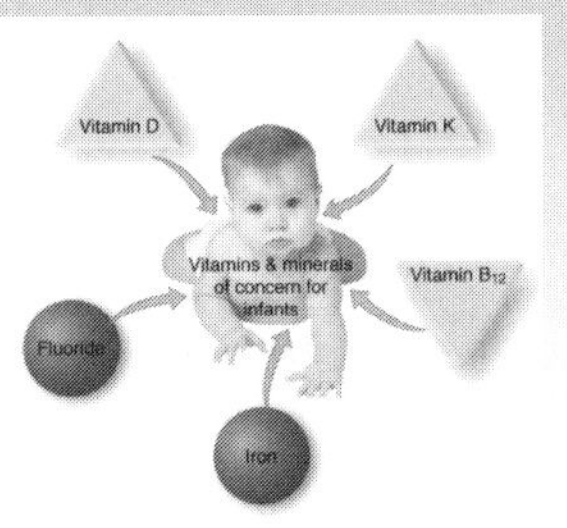

Photo © PhotoDisc

Introduction of Solid Foods

- Readiness for solids
  - Physiological readiness
    - Digestive enzymes
    - Ability to maintain hydration
  - Developmental readiness
    - Lack of extrusion reflex
    - Head and body control
- Feeding schedule
  - Start Healthy Feeding Guidelines (Table 12.20)

Feeding Problems During Infancy

- Colic
- Baby bottle tooth decay
- Iron-deficiency anemia
- Gastroesophageal reflux
- Diarrhea
- Failure to thrive

Notes

CHAPTER 13

Life Cycle: From Childhood through Adulthood

The chapter outline provides you with an organizational guide to the topics and ideas presented in this chapter of the text.

Key Terms

Define the following terms.

1. adolescence ______________________________

2. macular degeneration ______________________________

3. **menarche** ____________________

4. **urinary tract infection (UTI)** ____________________

5. **epiphyses** ____________________

6. **National School Lunch Program** ____________________

7. **hyperactivity** ____________________

8. **anorexia of aging** ____________________

9. **puberty** ____________________

10. **childhood** ____________________

◎ Fill-in-the-Blank

1. An inflammatory skin eruption that usually occurs in or near the sebaceous glands of the face, neck, shoulders, and upper back is ____________________.

2. The ____________________ is a USDA program that helps single people and families with little or no income to buy food.

3. The ____________________ is a federally funded program that provides older persons with nutritionally sound meals through meals-on-wheels programs or in senior citizen centers and similar congregate settings.

4. The ____________________ assists schools in providing a nutritious morning meal to children nationwide.

5. ____________________ is a presenile dementia characterized by accumulation of plaques in certain regions of the brain and degeneration of a certain class of neurons.

6. Households whose members take in enough calories but have diets of reduced quality that do not meet all daily nutritional requirements are ____________________.

7. The ____________________ helps children in lower income families to continue receiving nutritious meals during long school vacations when they do not have access to school lunch or breakfast.

8. ____________________ is a voluntary, not-for-profit organization established to provide nutritious meals to homebound people (regardless of age) so they may maintain their independence and quality of life.

9. High levels of vitamins in the blood, usually a result of excess supplement intake, are called ____________________.

10. The minimum amount of flavor that must be present for a taste to be detected is the ________________ ____.

◎ Fill-in-the-Blank Summaries

Childhood

During the childhood years, which are from 1 year of age to adolescence, a typical child will gain 5 pounds and grow 2–3 inches annually. The nutrient that is the hardest for children to get adequate amounts of in their diets is ________________________. In one study, upper income Caucasian toddlers were found to have low intakes of vitamins ___________ and ______________. One of the greatest barriers to a child receiving proper nutrition is poverty. WIC is designed to follow children through their fifth birthdays by providing vouchers for milk, eggs, cereal, juice, cheese, and peanut butter or dried beans. Many people do not use this program because they think it only provides for infants still drinking formula. In children over ________________, efforts to lower fat, saturated fat, and cholesterol intake may reduce risks of chronic diseases. This is supported by the American Heart Association, National Heart, Lung, and Blood Institute, and the AAP, but not all agencies advocate cutting fat from children's diets before adolescence. Childhood obesity is increasing at an alarming rate in the United States. The most popular strategy for treating childhood obesity is ____. Lead toxicity is a concern for children, especially in areas of poverty where lead sources tend to be higher. Lead toxicity can result in ________________________________.

Adolescents

Adolescence is defined as the time between the onset of puberty and adulthood. It is a time of great physical growth and development. A typical girl has achieved about ________________ percent of her adult height by menarche. On average, a boy will grow ____________________________ during puberty. ________________ is complete when the epiphyses close. Adolescent females should expect and be prepared to gain about ________________________________ pounds during puberty. By adulthood, a typical woman's body composition is ______________________ percent, and a man's is ____________________________ percent. The energy needs during puberty are higher than at any other time during life except ____________________________. Adolescents are often concerned with acne. Treatments for acne include two medications such as Retin-A and Accutane, which both contain vitamin A. Vitamin A in the diet does not have any effect on acne. Adolescents are known to frequently participate in behaviors that are incompatible with good health. Smoking tobacco is apt to ________________________ appetite; smoking marijuana is apt to _______________ appetite.

Staying Young While Growing Older

Today older people represent the fastest growing segment of the U.S. population. The size of the population of people 65 years old and older is expected to ___________________________ between 2000 and 2030. Until the 1990s health and nutrition surveys barely addressed the needs of late adulthood. Safe, deliberate, and modest weight loss can reduce cardiovascular risks for older, overweight people who are otherwise healthy. People who gain weight after age ______________________________________ have a significantly increased risk of developing cardiovascular disease. In addition, being overweight is associated with ________________________, ____, and some types of cancer. Elders often have low ___________________________________ status, which can lead to brittle bones. Sustaining mobility is an important aspect of healthy aging. Physiological functions that affect our mobility begin to decline at the age of ____________________.

Notes

Discovering Nutrition
Second Edition Paul Insel R. Elaine Turner Don Ross

Life Cycle: From Childhood Through Adulthood

Chapter 13

Childhood

- Energy and nutrient needs during childhood
  - Energy and protein
    - Kilocalories and grams protein per kg decrease from infancy
  - Vitamins and minerals
    - Variety of foods needed
    - Need for supplements?
- Influences on childhood food habits and intake

Nutritional Concerns of Childhood

- Malnutrition and hunger
- Food and behavior
- Nutrition and chronic disease
- Childhood overweight
- Lead toxicity
- Vegetarianism

Notes

Adolescence

- Physical growth and development
  - Adolescent growth spurt
    - Boys: begins between 12 and 13 years
      - Gain about 8 inches in height, 45 pounds in weight
    - Girls: begins between 10 and 11 years
      - Gain about 6 inches in height, 35 pounds in weight
    - Changes in body composition
    - Changes in emotional maturity

Nutrient Needs of Adolescents

- Energy and protein
  - Highest total calories and protein grams per day
- Vitamins and minerals

Influences on Adolescent Food Intake

Notes

Nutrition-Related Concerns for Adolescents

- Fitness and sports
- Acne
- Eating disorders
- Obesity
- Tobacco, alcohol, recreational drugs

Staying Young While Growing Older

- Age-related changes
  - Weight and body composition
    - Add fat, lose lean body mass
  - Mobility
    - Reduced muscle and skeletal strength
  - Immunity
    - Decline in defense mechanisms
  - Taste and smell
    - Decline in sensitivity
  - Gastrointestinal changes
    - Reduced acid secretion, reduced motility

Photo © PhotoDisc

Nutrient Needs of the Mature Adult

- Energy
  - Reduced needs
    - Decreased activity, decreased lean body mass
- Protein
  - Same needs per kg body weight as younger adults
- Carbohydrate
  - More likely to be lactose intolerant

Notes

Nutrient Needs of the Mature Adult

- Fat
  - Maintain moderate low-fat diet
- Water
  - Reduced thirst response

Nutrient Needs of the Mature Adult

- Vitamins of concern
  - Vitamin D
    - Needed for bone health, calcium balance
    - Reduced skin synthesis, activation
    - Higher needs
  - B vitamins
    - Reduced ability to absorb vitamin B_{12}
    - Folate, B_6, B_{12} may help reduce heart disease risk

Nutrient Needs of the Mature Adult

- Minerals of concern
  - Calcium
    - Bone health
    - Reduced ability to absorb calcium
  - Zinc
    - Marginal deficiencies likely
    - May compromise immunity, wound healing
  - Magnesium
  - Iron
    - Elders may have limited intake

Nutrition-Related Concerns of Mature Adults

- Drug-drug and drug-nutrient interactions
  - Can affect use of drugs or nutrients
- Depression
  - May reduce food intake
  - Alcoholism can interfere with nutrient use

Nutrition-Related Concerns of Mature Adults

- Anorexia of aging
  - Loss of appetite with illness
  - Can lead to protein-energy malnutrition
- Arthritis
  - May interfere with food preparation and eating
  - Dietary changes may improve symptoms

Nutrition-Related Concerns of Mature Adults

- Bowel and bladder regulation
  - Increased risk of urinary tract infection
  - Chronic constipation more common with age
    - Need for increased fluids, fiber
- Dental health
  - May interfere with eating ability, food choices

Notes

Notes

Nutrition-Related Concerns of Mature Adults

- Vision problems
  - Can affect ability to shop, cook
  - Antioxidants may reduce macular degeneration
- Osteoporosis
  - Common in elders, especially women
  - Maintain calcium, vitamin D, exercise

Nutrition-Related Concerns of Mature Adults

- Alzheimer's disease
  - Affects ability to function
  - Reduced taste, smell
  - Risk for weight loss, malnutrition

Meal Management for Mature Adults

- Managing independently
  - Services for elders
    - Meals on Wheels
    - Elderly Nutrition Program
    - Food Stamp Program

CHAPTER 14

Food Safety and Technology: Microbial Threats and Genetic Engineering

The chapter outline provides you with an organizational guide to the topics and ideas presented in this chapter of the text.

Food Safety
- Harmful Substances in Foods
- Keeping Food Safe
- Who's at Increased Risk for Foodborne Illness?
- A Final Word on Food Safety

Food Technology
- Food Preservation

Genetically Modified Foods
- A Short Course in Plant Genetics
- Genetically Modified Foods: An Unstoppable Experiment?
- Benefits of Genetic Engineering
- Risks
- Regulation

Key Terms

Define the following terms.

1. **irradiation** ______
2. **biodiversity** ______
3. **dioxins** ______
4. **pesticides** ______
5. **solanine** ______
6. **critical control points (CCPs)** ______
7. **organic foods** ______
8. **poisonous mushrooms** ______
9. **Food Code** ______
10. **prions** ______
11. **foodborne illness** ______

12. **Bt gene**____________________

13. **genome** ____________________

14. ***Salmonella*** ____________________

15. **methyl mercury** ____________________

16. **integrated pest management (IPM)**____________________

◎ Fill-in-the-Blank

1. ____________________ is a chronic degenerative disease, widely referred to as "mad cow disease," that affects the central nervous system of cattle.
2. ____________________ is a modern food safety system that focuses on preventing contamination by identifying potential areas in food production and retail in which contamination could occur and taking steps to ensure contaminants are not introduced at these points.
3. Bacteria that are the most common cause of urinary tract infections are ____________________. Because they release toxins, these bacteria can rapidly cause shock and death.
4. Foods produced using plant or animal ingredients that have been modified using gene technology are known as ____________________.
5. The ____________________ is a nonprofit organization devoted to increasing public awareness of food allergy and anaphylaxis (a life-threatening allergic reaction), educating the public about food allergies, and advancing research on food allergies.
6. ____________________ is a national organization devoted to preventing illness and death from foodborne illness by working with government agencies and industry to encourage practices and policies that promote safe food.
7. A process for destroying pathogenic bacteria by heating liquid foods to a prescribed temperature for a specified time is ____________________.
8. Chemicals or other agents that slow the decomposition of a food are ____________________.
9. ____________________ is a chemical produced in starchy foods by high-temperature cooking methods and found to be carcinogenic in animal tests.
10. ____________________ refers to the set of laboratory

techniques and processes used to modify the genome of plants or animals and thus create desirable new characteristics—genetic engineering in the broad sense.

11. ______________________________ is an often fatal type of food poisoning caused by a toxin released from *Clostridium botulinum,* a bacterium that can grow in improperly canned low-acid foods.

12. The ______________________________ was a 1996 presidential directive to three cabinet members to identify specific steps to improve the safety of the U.S. food supply.

13. A toxin found in more than 300 species of Caribbean and South Pacific fish, ______________ ______________ is a nonbacterial source of food poisoning.

14. Poisons that are produced by or naturally occur in plants or microorganisms are called ______________ ______________.

15. Manipulation of the genome of an organism by artificial means for the purpose of modifying existing traits or adding new genetic traits is called ______________ ______________.

16. Carcinogenic and toxic factors produced by food molds are ______________.

17. ______________________________ are gaseous, chemical, or organic wastes that contaminate air, soil, or water.

◎ Fill-in-the-Blank Summaries

Food Safety

Researchers at the CDC estimate that ______________ deaths are caused by foodborne illnesses each year. The seven most common foodborne pathogens are responsible for $6.5 to $34.9 billion in medical costs and lost productivity each year. Foodborne illnesses can result directly from infection with a ______________ or from the toxins it produces. ______________ ______________ is a bacterium that can grow in improperly canned low-acid foods. Choosing eggs cooked "over easy" could be disastrous because inadequate cooking can leave you vulnerable to ______________ ______________.

One way to avoid consuming the chemicals used in pesticides is to eat organic foods. Organic foods are grown without ______________. Products made with 50% to 95% organic ingredients can use the phrase ______________________________ on the label.

______________________________ are chemical compounds created in the manufacturing, combustion, and chlorine bleaching of pulp and paper. The FDA has concluded that these products pose no significant risk to human health because the quantity of this toxic chemical is minimal.

Food Technology

The most common antimicrobial agents used to preserve food are ________________ and ________________. Vitamin C and vitamin E can be used to preserve the color and flavor of foods that may be lost with exposure to air because they are ______________________________.

The FDA has approved food irradiation for ______________________________. Irradiation can reduce pathogens in raw poultry by as much as ________________ percent. Genetically modified foods are already available on the market. Genetic engineering allows scientists to transform a plant one gene at a time. ______________________ has/have been slow to accept genetically modified crops primarily because of ______________________________. The U.S. federal government has been ______________________________ of the trend toward GM food.

Notes

Discovering Nutrition
Second Edition Paul Insel R. Elaine Turner Don Ross

Food Safety and Technology: Microbial Threats and Genetic Engineering

Chapter 14

Food Safety

- Harmful substances in foods
  - Pathogens
    - Bacteria, viruses, parasites
  - Foodborne illness
    - Infection from pathogen
    - Toxin produced by microorganism

Food Safety

- Common causes of foodborne illness
  - *Staphylococcus aureus*
  - *Clostridium botulinum*
  - *Salmonella*
  - *Escherichia coli*

Notes

Food Safety

- Harmful substances in food
  - Chemical contamination
    - Pesticides
      - Organic alternatives
    - Animal drugs
    - Pollutants

Photo © PhotoDisc

Food Safety: Harmful Substances

- Natural toxins
  - Aflatoxins
  - Ciguatera
  - Methylmercury
  - Poisonous mushrooms
  - Solanine

Keeping Food Safe: Government Agencies

FSIS USDA Food Safety and Inspection Service
CSREES Cooperative State Research, Education, and Extension Service
ARS USDA Agricultural Research Service
EPA Environmental Protection Agency
CDC The Centers for Disease Control and Prevention
FDA Food and Drug Administration
Federal Food Safety

Keeping Food Safe: Food Industry

- Hazard Analysis Critical Control Point (HACCP): seven steps
  - Analyze hazards
  - Identify critical control points
  - Establish preventive measures with critical limits
  - Establish procedures to monitor control points
  - Establish corrective actions if critical limit isn't met
  - Establish effective record keeping
  - Establish procedures to verify that the system is working consistently

Keeping Food Safe: Consumer

- Clean
- Separate
- Cook
- Chill

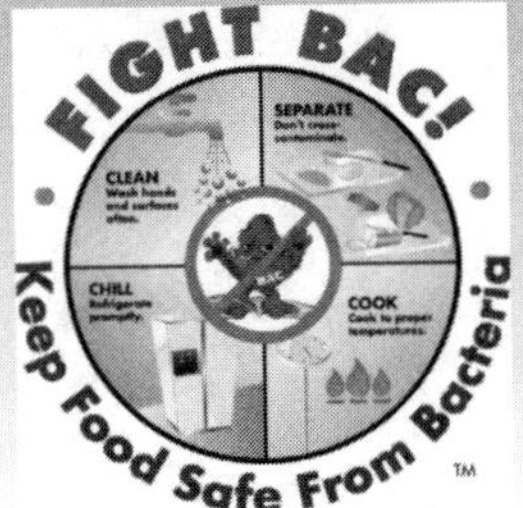

Clean: Wash hands and surfaces often
Separate: Don't cross-contaminate
Cook: Cook to proper temperatures
Chill: Refrigerate properly

Illustration courtesy of Partnership for Food Safety Education

Risk for Foodborne Illness

- Immune disorders
- Cancer
- Diabetes
- Long-term steroid use
- Liver disease
- Hemochromatosis
- Stomach problems

Notes

Notes

Food Technology

- Food preservation
  - Preservatives
    - Salt, sugar
    - Antioxidants
  - Other preservation techniques
    - Salting
    - Fermenting
    - Drying
    - Canning
    - Heating (e.g., pasteurization)
    - Irradiation

Preservatives

Pasteurization

Irradiation

Photos © Corbis Digital Images

Food Technology: Irradiation

FDA-APPROVED USES OF IRRADIATION

Approved foods Controls insects

Fruits and vegetables Delays maturation

Poultry Controls disease-causing microorganisms

Spices and dry vegetable seasonings Decontaminates and controls insects and microorganisms

Dry or dehydrated enzyme preparations Controls insects and microorganisms

Red meats (beef, lamb, pork) Controls spoilage and disease-causing microorganisms

Genetically Modified Foods

- Plant genetics
  - Traditional breeding
    - Cross two plants, develop hybrids; takes time
  - Genetic engineering
    - Transform specific genes
    - Less time needed to get desired effects

Red fruit with thin skin

Green fruit with thick skin

Red fruit with thick skin

Genetically Modified Foods

- Benefits of genetic engineering
  - Enhanced plant growth
  - Reduced pesticide and fertilizer use
  - Enhanced nutrient composition
  - Enhanced crop yields
- Risks
  - Potential for new allergens
  - Herbicide-resistant weeds
  - Loss of biodiversity

Genetically Modified Foods

- Regulation
  - FDA oversees genetically modified foods
  - Label requirements
    - If food is significantly different
    - If there are issues regarding use of the food
    - If food has different nutritional properties
    - If new food contains unexpected allergen

Notes

CHAPTER 15

World View of Nutrition: The Faces of Global Malnutrition

The chapter outline provides you with an organizational guide to the topics and ideas presented in this chapter of the text.

Malnutrition in the United States
- The Face of American Malnutrition
- Prevalence and Distribution
- Attacking Hunger in America

Malnutrition in the Developing World
- Why Hunger?
- Social and Economic Factors
- Infection and Disease
- Political Disruptions and Natural Disasters
- Inequitable Food Distribution
- Agriculture and Environment: A Tricky Balance
- Malnutrition: Its Nature, Its Victims, and Its Eradication

◎ Key Terms

Define the following terms.

1. **hunger** ________________________________
2. **food insecurity** ________________________________
3. **iodine deficiency disorders (IDD)** ________________________________
4. **Food Security Supplement Survey** ________________________________
5. **malnutrition** ________________________________
6. **Electronic Benefits Transfer (EBT)** ________________________________

◎ Fill-in-the-Blank

1. ________________________________ means having access to enough food for an active, healthy life, including (1) the ready availability of nutritionally adequate and safe foods and (2) an assured ability to acquire acceptable foods in socially acceptable ways.

2. The ______________________________ is a federally funded program that reimburses approved family child-care providers for USDA-approved foods served to preschool children; it also provides funds for meals and snacks served at after-school programs for school-age children and to adult day care centers serving chronically impaired adults or people over age 60.

3. The ______________________________ is a global organization that directs and coordinates international health work. Its goal is the attainment by all peoples of the highest possible level of health, defined as a state of complete physical, mental, and social well-being and not merely the absence of disease or infirmity.

4. The largest autonomous UN agency, the ______________________________, works to alleviate poverty and hunger by promoting agricultural development, improved nutrition, and the pursuit of food security.

5. The ______________________________ is a 1996 federal welfare reform plan that dramatically changed the nation's welfare system into one that requires work in exchange for time-limited assistance.

6. Founded in 1970 as a public interest law firm, the ______________________________ is a nonprofit child advocacy group that works to improve public policies to eradicate hunger and undernutrition in the United States.

Fill-in-the-Blank Summaries

Malnutrition in the United States

Paul, Sandy, and their two children have had hard times lately. Both Paul and Sandy lost their jobs in the past the year. They had a hard time finding new jobs and were forced to take high pay cuts in order to keep working. They have exhausted any back up funds they had saved and now slip into debt further from paycheck to paycheck. More of their budget now goes to their own food and less goes toward fixed expenses. This family is not alone in the United States. Almost __________ million households experienced hunger in the United States in 2003. Food insecurity is strongly associated with poverty. To be considered in poverty as a four member family, Paul and Sandy's joint income must be under ____________________; however, they are considered part of the working poor and are therefore eligible for benefits under the ______________________________.

Malnutrition: Its Nature, Its Victims, and Its Eradication

Hunger is a global problem. Despite gains in eradicating malnutrition, __________ percent of the people in the developing world continue to suffer from chronic hunger. Although world food supplies are adequate, factors that allow hunger to continue include ______________, ______________, and ______________________. Infection, especially ______________________________, rapid population growth, and other factors threaten to reverse hard-won gains. The most critical nutrition deficiencies in today's developing world include ______________________, ______________________, and ______________________. Fortification and supplementation programs are effectively attacking iodine and vitamin A deficiencies but have less success overcoming ______________________ deficiency. ______________________ of the underlying causes of malnutrition must be addressed to reduce and eliminate these and other deficiencies.

Notes

Discovering Nutrition
Second Edition Paul Insel R. Elaine Turner Don Ross

World View of Nutrition: The Faces of Global Malnutrition

Chapter 15

A Few Definitions

- Hunger
  - Uneasy or painful sensation caused by lack of food
- Malnutrition
  - Failure to achieve nutrient requirements
- Food insecurity
  - Limited or uncertain availability of nutrients or food
- Food security
  - Access to enough food

Malnutrition in the United States

- Prevalence and distribution
  - Linked with economic and social factors

PREVALENCE OF FOOD INSECURITY

Key
Below national average
Near national average
Above national average

Malnutrition in the United States: Groups at Risk

- Working poor
  - May or may not qualify for food assistance
- Isolated
  - Lack access to food resources
- Elders
  - Economic difficulties
  - Physical ailments

Malnutrition in the United States: Groups at Risk

- Homeless
  - Lack consistent cooking facilities
  - Limited income, if any
- Children
  - Dependent on family circumstances
  - Hunger affects school performance

Malnutrition in the United States

- Attacking hunger in America
  - The Food Stamp program
    - Extends food buying power
  - Special Supplemental Nutrition Program for Women, Infants, and Children (WIC)
    - Food and nutrition services for pregnant and lactating women, and children to age 5
  - National School Lunch Program
    - Free and reduced-price meals
  - Child and Adult Care Food Program

Notes

Notes

Malnutrition in the Developing World

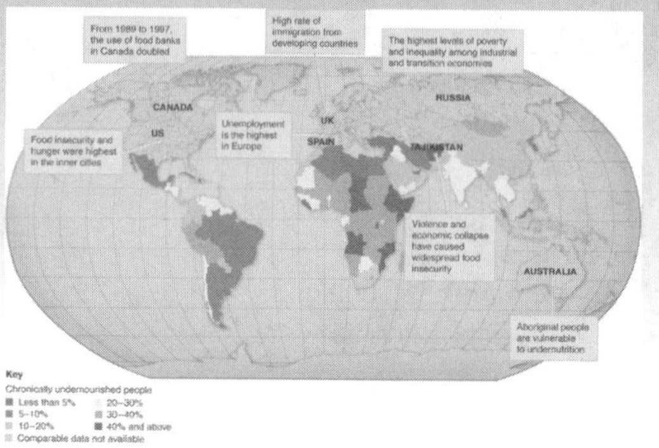

Malnutrition in the Developing World

- Factors that contribute to hunger and malnutrition
  - Social and economic factors
    - Poverty
    - Population growth
    - Urbanization

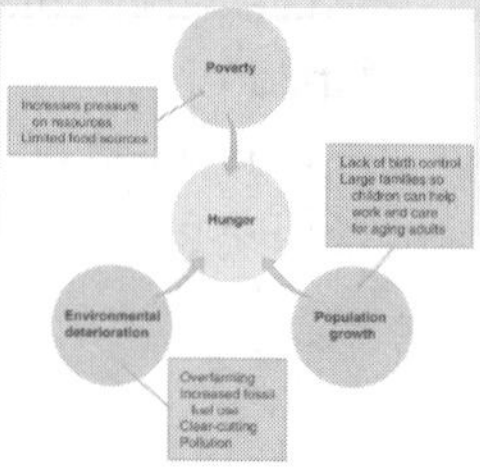

Malnutrition in the Developing World

- Factors that contribute to hunger and malnutrition
  - Infection and disease
  - Political disruptions and natural disasters
    - War
    - Refugees
    - Sanctions
    - Floods, droughts, mudslides, hurricanes
  - Inequitable food distribution

Malnutrition in the Developing World

- Agriculture and environment: a tricky balance
  - Environmental degradation
    - Reduced food production
    - Nutritional consequences

Malnutrition in the Developing World

- Kwashiorkor
- Marasmus

Malnutrition in the Developing World

- Iodine deficiency disorders
  - Most common cause of preventable brain damage

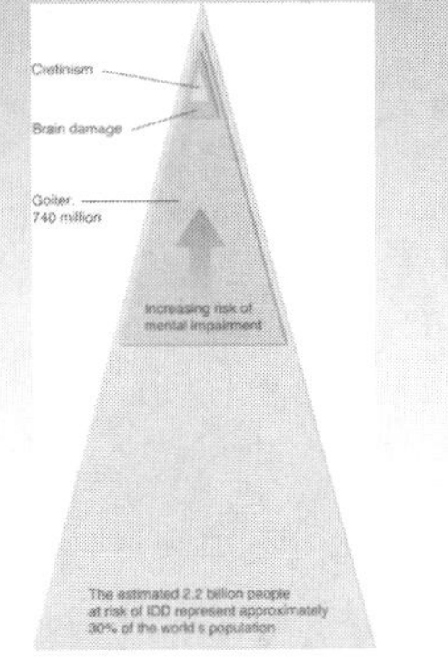

Notes

Notes

Malnutrition in the Developing World

- Vitamin A deficiency
  - Leading cause of preventable blindness
- Iron-deficiency anemia
  - Limits productivity of population

Malnutrition in the Developing World

- Other vitamin, mineral deficiencies
- Overweight and obesity
  - Differing cultural attitudes
  - High-calorie, low-nutrient-dense foods